"It takes courage to step into the maelstrom of groups blaming groups. Individual hurts and trauma lead to blame, shame and guilt, but when the large group is involved, morality, meaning and transgenerational transmission add fuel to the fire and we are all in danger of getting burnt. This book takes us along a path we need to tread in the cause of survival. It is a book that leaves a lasting message in your mind and I strongly recommend it."

John Alderdice, FRCPsych, The Changing Character of War Centre, Pembroke College, Oxford

"We live in an era when individuals pride themselves on their victim status, grievances are carefully nurtured, public apologies are *de rigueur* and reparations are constantly demanded of the formerly powerful. Covington's book cuts to the chase, subjecting our modern blame culture to forensic examination. She questions whether apologies of this sort make logical, historical or legal sense and what therapeutic emotional value they actually possess. A welcome breath of fresh, bracing air."

Michela Wrong, author of *Do Not Disturb: The Story of a Political Murder and a Regime Gone Bad*

"In this brilliant study of collective guilt, Coline Covington fuses together the disciplines of history, politics, and psychoanalysis, helping us to understand the profound effects of blame on perpetrators and victims across generations. Her writing is both lucid and learned throughout."

Charles Grant, Director, Centre for European Reform

T0172391

Who's to Blame? Collective Guilt on Trial

Who's to Blame? Collective Guilt on Trial presents a psychoanalytic exploration of blame and collective guilt in the aftermath of large-scale atrocities that cause widespread trauma and victimization.

Coline Covington explores various aspects of social and collective guilt and considers how both perpetrators and victims make sense of their experiences, with particular reference to group behavior and political morality. Covington challenges the concept of collective guilt associated with the aftermath of large-scale atrocities such as the Holocaust and examines the moral pressure placed on perpetrators to exhibit guilt as part of a realignment of political power and a process of restoring social morality. *Who's to Blame? Collective Guilt on Trial* concludes with a chapter-length case study examining Russia's war in Ukraine.

Combining psychoanalytic ideas with political, philosophical and social theory, *Who's to Blame? Collective Guilt on Trial* will be of great value to readers interested in questions of collective guilt, blame and the possibilities of atonement. It will also appeal to psychoanalysts in practice and in training, and to academics of psychoanalytic studies, political philosophy, sociology and conflict resolution.

Coline Covington has for many years combined her background in political science and criminology with her psychoanalytic practice and thinking. She is currently a Fellow of International Dialogue Initiative (IDI), a think tank on political conflict. She previously worked as a consultant to local authorities on juvenile justice policy and set up the first victim/offender mediation scheme in the UK with the Metropolitan Police. *Who's to Blame? Collective Guilt on Trial* is the third book of a trilogy on political morality.

Who's to Blame? Collective Guilt on Trial

Coline Covington

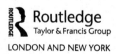

Routledge
Taylor & Francis Group

LONDON AND NEW YORK

First published 2023
by Routledge
4 Park Square, Milton Park, Abingdon, Oxon OX14 4RN

and by Routledge
605 Third Avenue, New York, NY 10158

Routledge is an imprint of the Taylor & Francis Group, an informa business

© 2023 Coline Covington

British Library Cataloguing-in-Publication Data
A catalogue record for this book is available from the British Library

ISBN: 978-1-032-46079-6 (hbk)
ISBN: 978-1-032-46078-9 (pbk)
ISBN: 978-1-003-37998-0 (ebk)

DOI: 10.4324/9781003379980

Typeset in Times New Roman
by Taylor & Francis Books

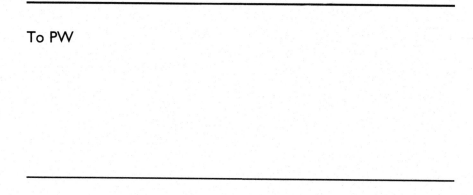

To PW

Contents

A scapegoat remains effective as long as we believe in its guilt.
(Rene Girard, 2009[1])

Acknowledgements

I would like to thank the many friends and colleagues who have seen my book through from conception to birth and have helped to clarify and deepen my thinking throughout. Special thanks go to Patricia Williams, Richard Carvalho and Owen Renik who have been critical and encouraging readers, and who have kept me company during my journey and tempered the isolation of writing. Thanks also to Charles Bland, Regine Scholz, Paul Rock and Jonathan Maynard Leader, who in the course of many discussions have contributed invaluable insights and perspectives. I would also like to thank my colleague, Lois Oppenheim, who has invited me for many years to preview my work at NYPSI public events. In addition, Hattie Myers, editor of the magazine ROOM, has promoted my writing and been an inspiration to work with. I am grateful to the members of International Dialogue Initiative who continue to nourish and stimulate my interest in political psychology. As always, Ted Jacobs is a guiding star of encouragement and friendship.

I would like to thank my patients who have courageously fought against blame and who have given me so much understanding. Their words, anonymized, open each chapter of this book.

Lastly, I thank Susannah Frearson at Routledge who has been wonderfully facilitating and a pleasure to work with.

Preface

I spent the first years of my life in North Carolina and Florida, where both my parents' families had come from. My first, and most beloved, nanny was a black woman called Beulah, who was as close to a mother as I had. Throughout the south and in many other countries where childcare was assigned to servants, or in some instances, to virtual slaves, this relationship was of fundamental importance and inevitably complicated in its nature.

My family had been amongst the original settlers from England establishing landholdings in the south, many of which were to become plantations and many of these ultimately supported by slaves. Slaves were not, as is often thought to be the case, initially money-making for the plantations. They became an increasingly expensive financial drain as their upkeep became more costly than their productivity – until the invention of the cotton mill, which transformed the economy of the south and suddenly created a demand for cheap labor. Slavery boomed, and the inhuman treatment of blacks went largely unchecked, as black lives, particularly unproductive ones, became increasingly expendable in the marketplace.

I was aware as a child that all the servants of my extended family were black. They lived in poor conditions in the poor part of town and, by and large, they were devoted to my family – or certainly seemed so. There was a postbellum system of *noblesse oblige* in which many white southern families continued in some ways to care for the black people whose parents and grandparents had been their slaves. Basic healthcare, clothing, housing, and care in emergencies for the family servants were frequently discussed as being the automatic duty of the family. This is not to paint a rosy picture of black lives in the first half of the twentieth century. Racism was embedded in the culture, and real opportunities for black people to improve their social position were minimal and required extraordinary perseverance and courage. Nevertheless, my parents considered themselves liberal, they supported black rights movements, and were the first to criticize slavery as a crime against humanity.

Against this backdrop, my family moved north to New York City when I was four years old, and my life changed in some ways beyond recognition. We no longer had servants, I was no longer cared for by Beulah, I had to translate my mother's southern drawl to the local shopkeepers who thought she came from a foreign country, and I could no longer run free in our tropical garden filled with lemons, limes, coconuts, quince, pineapples and avocadoes that I could pick up from the ground as they ripened. In New York, while my father went to work at his office every day, my mother was isolated and depressed, and I felt a deep homesickness that has in some way never left me – a homesickness for place and for the warmth of extended family, and especially for the servants I loved who had taken care of me and on whom I had depended.

This is a typical portrait of nostalgia that many people who have been uprooted can relate to. But it was also to become tinged with the family history of the American Civil War and its devastation to the lives of many in the south – both the rich families, and the poor who depended on the rich for their livelihoods. The common topic of conversation at my family breakfast table on Sunday mornings was what happened in the war; stories of loss and bitterness when everything that families had worked for had been destroyed, stories of young and old men, distant relatives, slaughtered on the battlefields – and of beloved slaves who died defending their owners. And stories of the survivors: traumatized and emasculated men turning to drink, hard-pressed women taking over farmsteads and the running of the family, and newly freed slaves who could barely subsist. The wounds inflicted by civil war are far deeper than wars fought on foreign soil and, in most societies, are marked by a generation of men, physically and emotionally crippled, and of women forced by default into the role of the head of the family. A matriarchy founded on loss and violence.

In my family's new life in New York, we employed a black cleaning lady who my mother helped out in a number of ways when she could, financially and otherwise. My mother made it clear that this was because we were relatively privileged and, as such, we had an obligation to help others who were not as well off. This was not a religious belief – my parents were not especially religious – but part of one's social responsibility. I remember, however, that my mother would comment on the fact that this attitude was not shared by many other housewives she encountered in the north. Whether or not this was because of my mother's southern background is a moot point. What was clear was that the idea of guilt was never mentioned by either of my parents. Although both my parents came from slaveholding families and both abhorred slavery, neither of them ever talked about their past with a sense of guilt or shame for that matter. It was the past and not of their making.

The real wound that had traumatized my entire family and much of the white southern population had been the Civil War; this was certainly transmitted to me over the breakfast table. My father's fantasies, bizarrely unreal in retrospect, of how our lives might have been if the south had won or if the war had never occurred colored my view of the south and fed an underlying and still present antagonism towards the north, who were seen as the perpetrators. Even discounting the fantasies, the war had created a deep rupture in people's lives that was still alive and raw at our family breakfast table a hundred years later, overshadowing some of the broader issues of the Civil War.

Although my family's ruin was all in the past, the trauma of the war and the massive losses that it inflicted throughout the south left deep scars amongst many of the white families who had suffered badly – scars that were passed on from one generation to the next in the form of bitterness, prejudice and the abusiveness that comes from humiliation and defeat. For black people, many of whom were better off, freedom had not made a significant difference to the institutionalized racism that permeated southern society and, it is important to add, northern society as well. In my own family, blame was clearly placed at the doorstep of the northern Unionists, who were seen as having no understanding of southern culture and who were depicted as the greedy industrialists who were threatening a whole way of life. These deep divisions in the US are still very much alive even if their geography has changed.

As I grew up, historical analysis and interpretation of the American Civil War changed according to fashion and political correctness, something that is still happening in today's history telling. There were two key opposing lines of argument – that the basis of the war had been economic versus that the basis was about emancipation. The reality is that both are true, but the issue of emancipation did not take center stage until towards the end of the war when the north was clearly losing, the casualties were immense and it was increasingly hard to recruit soldiers for a cause that was of little relevance to the common man and mostly of benefit to the rich industrialists of the north.

President Lincoln's Emancipation Proclamation, delivered on 1st January 1863, significantly reframed the war as a battle for freedom, not a battle to preserve the Union. In his documentary series on the Civil War, Ken Burns quotes from the diary of John Hay, the President's 23-year-old secretary:

> At a Washington dinner … everyone seemed to feel a new sort of exhilarating life. The President's proclamation had freed them, as well as the slaves …. It was no longer a question of the union as it was that was to be re-established, it was the union as it should be, that is to say, washed clean from its original sin. We were no longer merely the soldiers of a political controversy, we were now the missionaries of a great work of redemption, the armed liberators of millions. The war was ennobled. The object was higher …

This slice of history reminds us that political rationales, perhaps especially in relation to war, alter with changing circumstances and are molded according to what is considered politically acceptable at any given time. The history of the war in Viet Nam is a particularly apposite example of this. For many in the south, including my family, this revision of the cause of the Civil War came as an afterthought and was not central to what most southerners thought they were fighting for. It is an example of what we can think of as a "chosen narrative" that is linked to an event and subsequently connected to what the founder of political psychology, Vamik Volkan, describes as a "chosen trauma".

Lincoln's reframing of the war firmly positioned the north as representing the superior, righteous cause while condemning the south as immoral and impure. The battle was, indeed, against original sin itself. Harking back to the Declaration of Independence, emancipation of the slaves also formed the next logical step in the history of liberation from an elite ruling class and, as such, was in complete accordance with the democratic principles upon with the United States was founded. Freedom for all is worth dying for. From this "chosen narrative", follows the "chosen trauma", selectively framed by the winners of the war. While the trauma of slavery cannot be diminished, the chosen trauma takes precedence and obfuscates the traumas experienced by others, in this case the trauma of a civil war that pits families against each other and leaves lasting memories of violence.

My experience within my own family is not so dissimilar to many others whose fortunes have suddenly been reversed and, most notably, who are branded by their past. The obvious analogy is with Germany after the fall of the Third Reich. The moral philosopher, Susan Neiman, in her book, *Learning from the Germans*, draws on the efforts of post-war Germany to atone for its past as an exemplar of what other large groups responsible for crimes against other racial groups should do. While I would argue that it is important for us to remember what crimes we are capable of committing and how terrifyingly easy it is to slip into evil, Neiman takes a moral position that the group retains not just collective responsibility for its past but collective guilt. I will in later chapters challenge this position, but I mention it here because it is an argument that has, since my childhood, always come across as conferring on me what I "should" feel without any recognition of the reality of my experience and the experience of others, and our relationship to our own family and collective histories.

Our view of history, whether it is our own personal history or our collective history, is most often based on causal, sequential narratives that explain why things happened the way they did and, most importantly, who within this narrative are the heroes and who are the villains – who made things good again and who are the ones to blame. The moral tenets of our Judeo-Christian tradition are derived in part from this archetypal narrative that we construct of the world and that also perpetuates a binary view of events and how we "should" understand and feel about them.

Just as I do not want to be told to forgive someone who has viciously hurt me, I do not want to be told that I am guilty of my ancestors' crimes. This does not mean I am not responsible for myself and my actions in the present. But these moral dictates stop us from thinking and from questioning our own experience. How large groups of people "should" feel can be a dangerous mechanism of political control and manipulation, distorting our view of the world, our past and our very psyches. Without understanding the blindness of our forebears and how they were able to live with and perpetrate cruelty towards other humans, we risk ignoring our blindness in the present. Expressing guilt about the collective wrongdoings of our ancestors may give us some sense of redemption or social cleansing in the present, but it does not change the past nor does it necessarily change our actions in the present. It is a moral and political gesture that identifies perpetrators and victims within a framework of chosen trauma that can then be used to perpetuate hatred of the "other" while establishing the righteousness of others not involved. Our duty to ourselves and to our children is to situate our chosen traumas as events that can help us to understand how atrocities occur – within every human society and within every individual. Understanding how we become complicit in atrocities is not the same thing as condoning them – but it is a far more effective prophylactic than guilt.

Note

1 This quotation originally appeared in Rene Girard, *Battling to the End: Conversations With Benoit Chantre,* 2009, published by Michigan State University Press.

Introduction

Since the COVID-19 pandemic, the question of the state's moral and social responsibility for its citizens has come to the forefront of our political consciousness. The balance between preserving people's lives and salvaging the world economy has perhaps never been so starkly challenged. Poor leadership that has led to mishandling of both healthcare and economic interests has triggered deeper inequalities, and social divisions are surfacing with a vengeance. The greatest of these is the Black Lives Matter protest that has now spread worldwide and has brought in its wake a re-questioning of history, how history is depicted in the present and the historical injustices that continue to beleaguer the fabric of our society and form much of the basis for ongoing inequality. The oppression of one race by another – and the consequences of this – raise further questions about collective guilt. For example, should white Americans today acknowledge and atone for the guilt of their slaveholding fathers? How much do we expect any racial or political group to plead guilty to the harm their predecessors have done to others in the past and, if we do expect this, how can it be expressed in any meaningful and moral way? Does collective guilt extend to the destructiveness and deaths incurred in warfare and, if not, how do we draw a line between what is excessive and what is morally acceptable? These are the questions that *Who's to Blame?* addresses through the lens of history, recent events and individual case histories from my psychoanalytic practice.

My book looks at collective guilt on a broad social basis in the aftermath of large-scale atrocities[1] that have caused widespread trauma and victimization. I am using the term "collective guilt" here as distinct from "collective responsibility"; while a large group may be responsible for actions that harm another group and in this regard may be considered guilty, it does not follow that all members of the group experience guilt, or that subsequent generations can be held accountable for the actions of their forebears. The moral pressure placed on perpetrators to exhibit guilt is understood in this context as part of a realignment of political power and a process of restoring social morality. This does not mean, however, that large groups necessarily feel guilty or behave accordingly. I explore different aspects of social and collective guilt, and how both perpetrators and victims respond and make sense of their

DOI: 10.4324/9781003379980-1

experiences in different ways according to their different situations. For example, immediately after the end of World War Two, following Hitler's suicide, there was a wave of suicides across Germany, often mistakenly attributed to guilt when in fact there were many other more powerful factors at work, such as terror of Russian reprisals. Our Judeo-Christian expectation that perpetrators should feel guilty and atone for their crimes colors our political relationships and creates moral splits that can exacerbate rather than help in healing the after-effects of violence. Even when guilt may be genuinely acknowledged within a country, this is not an antidote to xenophobia and racism that we see re-emerging across Europe and elsewhere. In Rwanda, for example, although President Kagame has restored social order, old hatreds lie dormant beneath the surface and threaten to re-surface when Kagame is no longer in power. The Black Lives Matter movement highlights the fact that racism and historical persecution are structurally rooted and perpetuated even in the face of government policies that attempt to rectify racist injustices.

This book is a companion to two previous books of mine that examine the belief systems and the political morality of large group behavior from a psychoanalytic perspective. The first book, *Everyday Evils: A Psychoanalytic View of Evil and Morality* (Routledge 2017), argues that atrocities, committed by seemingly ordinary people, arise out of belief systems that have become perverted but are based on our most powerful human need to belong and not to be outcast. This basic belief system also inspires, on the other hand, acts of bravery and patriotism, the subject of my second book, *For Goodness Sake: Bravery, Patriotism and Identity* (Phoenix Publishing House 2020). This third book questions the validity of the concept of collective guilt, arguing that it is largely a moral construct used politically to determine power relations. In conclusion, I question a basic assumption that runs through political analyses, regardless of their theoretical perspective, that groups behave similarly to individuals – or that they ought to – and argue that if this were so, history would not repeat itself.

I start my exploration of blame and collective guilt by looking at our natural proclivity to find someone to blame when something goes wrong, when there is a loss or injury of any kind, even when it may be clear that no one is responsible. Identifying someone to blame is an important means of making sense of our lives and, in particular, our suffering. The person who has been attacked or robbed wants to find the culprit in order to set things right again, to restore justice and a world of moral order. Blame also assumes a certain degree of agency on the part of the offender and this assures us some sense of control over our world. Notably it is always another country that either starts a war or provokes one's own country into aggression. Even in the case of natural disasters that are clearly beyond our control, we look for someone to blame. Identifying who is to blame is important not only in terms of punishment and restoration but more significantly as a way of understanding and accounting for a collective experience that has been chaotic and destructive. The more extreme the destructiveness, the greater the need to apportion blame.

In the case of atrocities, such as the Holocaust, blame is often targeted at the leader. Although as leader of the Third Reich, Hitler held ultimate responsibility for the Final Solution, what about all the other state officials and citizens who knowingly went along with this? Hannah Arendt was amongst the first writers and philosophers at that time to question collective morality and responsibility, propounding the view that, existentially, we are all to blame. This was also echoed by Primo Levi in his writing. If we accept this argument, then we are all collectively guilty because we are all part of humanity. However, our need to blame someone else and to exonerate ourselves remains a powerful political and social force that shapes our relations with other countries and within our own countries. Since the Holocaust, and atrocities committed in other parts of the world, moral pressure has been put on groups identified as perpetrators to admit to their crimes and, in doing so, to perform an act of social cleansing. This dynamic has recently surfaced in the far left in the US, as white people are held accountable for the sins of their slaveholding fathers.

The inheritance of guilt operates not only on a collective level but haunts those individuals whose parents and family members have been implicated in large-scale atrocities. How do you live with the knowledge that your father ordered the death of thousands of innocent people? Children of parents who have committed or been involved in atrocities have to live with the guilt of their parents' deeds, even when guilt is acknowledged by the parents. Because of their family history, these children often become "lightning conductors" for social guilt, tainted with the mark of evil and carrying blame for deeds they had nothing to do with In my second chapter, drawing on clinical material and interviews with children of Nazi SS officers, I examine the personal psychological repercussions and conflicts that children of perpetrators face in their lives.[2] These conflicts live on not only within the children who have inherited their parents' crimes but within the larger society in the form of memory, denial and guilt. The psychological dilemma for children of perpetrators provides a prism through which we can better understand the impact of past atrocities on the collective. The more profound role of shame experienced by these children and their families is also distinguished from guilt.

The following third chapter addresses the question of how collective guilt is ascribed and the consequent difficulty in administering some form of punishment. In Judeo-Christian culture, the confession and atonement for committing sins brings us back to God and restores social purity. Prior to the Holocaust, there are, across the world, many historical examples of atrocities committed on racial groups under the power of foreign empires or in the commercial enterprise of slavery. The Holocaust marked a turning point in the world's moral consciousness, bringing about the use of the word "genocide" and its meaning. For the first time in history, war crimes were viewed in a different light. The Nuremberg Trials held after the end of World War Two initiated legal recognition of individuals responsible for war crimes and crimes against humanity. Subsequent trials in Germany and the institution of the International Criminal Court of Justice at The Hague continue to hold individuals accountable for war crimes. These tribunals, however, do not determine the collective guilt of a nation.

If we look at postwar Germany as an example, the liberation of the concentration camps by the Allies was almost concurrently followed by Allied programs aimed at inducing guilt and shame in the German population. Queues of German citizenry were filmed as they were forced by the Allies to enter the camps and to witness the sites of mass killing. These programs were a clear expression of the moral imperative imposed on the German population from the Allies that they should take on the mantle of guilt as a nation for the evils that had been committed under the Reich.

While the Allies did not question the "rightness" of pointing the finger of collective guilt at the Germans, and indeed many Germans today agree on the importance of atoning for their guilt, the historical evidence of the German population experiencing actual guilt is complex and arguable. This also applies to other countries, such as Poland, Rwanda and Serbia, in which public displays of mourning over genocidal killings take on different meanings depending on the political and historical context.

Contrary to blaming others, the idea of collective guilt may serve to "normalize" what has happened and to protect the group from being tainted by evil. The experience and proximity of evil is contaminating and disorienting; it is also alienating. Above all, it is shameful. Guilt absolves the criminal – it reintegrates the criminal within "normal" society. The experience of shame is markedly different: shame stays within us and cannot be washed away. In Chapter Four I argue that shame is often mistaken for guilt but the two are in fact distinctly different with different effects on the individual and the group. This distinction is highlighted by Primo Levi's description of the shame experienced by the Russian soldiers as they liberated Auschwitz and became aware of the extreme atrocities that had taken place.

Levi recognizes that whoever witnesses a crime shares responsibility – merely in being human – for what has happened. We are linked through our deeds whether we like it or not. Levi also declares that the Germans running the concentration camps never knew shame. This was not because they weren't human but, perhaps most significantly, they were operating within a world of violence that was not only sanctioned but positively valued – a world in which they themselves had become dehumanized, in which they had allowed themselves to be used as tools of the state in achieving its ends and in their hope for a better future.

The difference between guilt and shame has important political repercussions. Guilt is associated with self-agency and arises from committing an act that is prohibited. As such, although groups can commit criminal acts, it is the individual who is ultimately accountable. Shame applies to one's being rather than to a specific act and is closely related to the emotion of disgust. Shame strips the individual and the group of honor and respect; the fundamental being of a person is de-humanized. By focusing on collective guilt, rather than shame, in the wake of atrocity, are we attempting to humanize something that is intrinsically de-humanizing?

As shame is such a profoundly painful experience, the most common way of combatting it is to try to hide what is perceived as shameful and to present an untarnished face to the world. In my fifth chapter, I argue that saving face is an important aspect of group identity and rests in each case on a particular construction of the group's history. Professor Vamik Volkan, psychoanalyst and founder of political psychology, coined the term "chosen trauma" to connote a mental representation of a massive trauma shared by a large group over generations to consolidate group identity and to establish the group's historical narrative. Alongside the "chosen trauma" is also the "chosen glory" that celebrates the strength of the group and bolsters self-esteem. When the group's existence is threatened, its chosen trauma is reactivated as a warning of danger and to instill aggression against the foreign enemy. Although the "chosen trauma" serves to strengthen group identity in times of crisis, it may have destructive consequences if it is used to reframe and distort history for political purposes. What is memorialized and what is vilified in a country's history, especially in relation to war, civil and otherwise, shape its identity and future relations with others, particularly in establishing which groups are considered "good" and which "bad". The debate in the US about Civil War memorials is a case in point, as is the heated debate in the UK that has led to the deposition of the Cecil Rhodes statue at Oxford University.

In attempting to deny involvement in atrocities, groups may also defend themselves by adopting the narrative that they were the real victims, either of an invading force or of prior historical conflicts. In common language, they shift the blame to someone else. When the aggressors are attacked, they become the wounded innocent and guilt is projected on to the other. The "chosen trauma" signifies the group as victim, not as aggressor, and absolves the group of wrongdoing. This process is apparent across cultures and time. In his famous address to the Reichstag on 1st September 1933 declaring the start of World War Two, Hitler accuses the Poles of attacking German territory. He goes a step further to declare that as the enemy "departs from the rules of human warfare", so will Germany in self-defense. Guilt is projected on to the other to maintain purity of the group. More recently, this process is also apparent in Poland's edict establishing that it had nothing to do with the atrocities committed on Polish soil.

Both "chosen traumas" and "chosen victories" are fundamental cornerstones of large group identity. Their centrality, however, also means that blame against the group is avoided and blame against the other is perpetuated. We advocate the importance of learning from history, especially after extreme violence, but it is the very dynamics of group identity that prevents us from learning from our past.

The difficulty in applying the same psychological framework of individual development to group behavior also becomes apparent in efforts to heal and absolve the group from guilt. In Chapter Six, I question the effectiveness of healing rituals and whether they are in fact misconceived, resulting in perpetuating a culture of blame rather than achieving some form of absolution.

Judeo-Christian cultures turn to rituals to acknowledge guilt, to seek forgiveness and to make atonement. These rituals are meant to restore moral order and to cleanse the group of hatred. Truth and reconciliation commissions, restorative justice and reparation have been the most common and widespread rituals of the twentieth century to come out of this moral tradition. Much hope was placed that these processes would create stronger and safer communities and that long-lasting peace could be established. However, as attempts to change group behavior, they have largely failed. A central problem is that they are based on a binary understanding of good and evil – rather than helping to contain conflict within a group. This approach only serves to create further psychological splitting, to delineate an us-them mentality even more sharply and to establish a moral high ground that reinforces political superiority. It also treats large groups as if they are individuals acting out of one will and one agency. In contrast to healing rituals, acts of revenge are not only natural responses to being attacked but they serve the important role of restoring a sense of agency and identity to the individual and to the victimized group. This is its strength but revenge also fuels counter-revenge and the cycle continues unless, as Machiavelli recommends, the injury is so great the enemy is unable to take revenge.

After acts of extreme violence that affect large groups, there are inevitably deep grievances – often on both sides. Chapter Seven examines the important role of apology in achieving some closure on long-standing conflicts and grievances. When leaders apologize for the harm their country has incurred on others it is a profound moment of acknowledgment that can salve the wounds of the past. We recall Willy Brandt in 1970 silently falling to his knees at the memorial service commemorating the Jewish victims of the Warsaw Ghetto, we have witnessed Queen Elizabeth admitting in her historic Dublin speech in 2011 the "sad and regrettable mistakes of Britain's troubled relationship with Ireland", five years later we saw Obama speaking out against the nuclear devastation at Hiroshima, and there are many other leaders and other apologies. These acknowledgments are perhaps most important as public markers of a history that cannot be denied or ignored. They set the record straight. But does this imply collective guilt?

In his preface to Dostoyevsky's *The Brothers Karamazov*, Freud wrote, "… the invading barbarians who killed and then did penance, penance thus becoming a technique permitting murder." Freud identifies the perverse aspect of atonement that allows the sinner to become righteous and then to continue to commit sins under the banner of righteousness. We are seeing today in those countries that have publicly made atonement for the persecution and killing of racial groups, e.g., Germany, South Africa and Rwanda, a resurfacing of racial hatred and xenophobia. This necessarily brings into question not only the efficacy of public atonement but whether it is in fact morally authentic or appropriate within the context of large group dynamics. It also raises the question as to whether we can apply the concept of mourning to large groups, especially when there is an incongruence in how loss is perceived and experienced. While it is important to uphold a certain moral code within society and to restore a belief in justice, collective gestures of atonement and memorialization may inadvertently create a false sense of unification that can prevent governments from seeing old conflicts re-emerging. Atonement does not by itself protect against the return of the repressed and it may in some instances even exacerbate it.

The important yet complicated role of atonement raises further questions about the place and effectiveness of social rituals. For example, do we need to find new rituals that are less fixed on laying blame but more effective at peace-keeping; rituals that help us to understand and acknowledge the hatred and violence that has occurred and often continues to exist, rituals that can help us to acknowledge conflicts without acting them out through violence, and, finally, rituals that do not stigmatize a group of people and in doing so create the same mistake as the perpetrators? Do we need to find rituals that bring us together in our mutual shame and loss rather than rituals that tear us apart in guilt?

Chapter Eight brings the reader up to date with an examination of Russia's invasion of Ukraine on 24th February 2022. Russia's attack on Ukraine highlights the central part that blame has played in the dynamics of the war as well as raising further questions about collective guilt and responsibility. While the United States and other Western countries view the war as a battle for the life of democracy, Putin has framed the invasion very differently as a battle to reinstate Ukraine within Russia where it had always belonged. In 2012, two years prior to the invasion of Crimea, Putin announced his intention to restore the boundaries of the Russian empire and to create a "historic future", a future based on the pure Russian culture as described in the writings of the Russian philosopher, Ivan Ilyin, and the ethnologist, Lev Gumilev. With the dissolution of the Soviet Republic and the demise of socialist ideology, Russia has experienced years of what can be described as a political ideological vacuum. Over his years in office, Putin has promoted a mythological narrative, represented in Gumilev's word "passionarnost", that guides his actions and is presented to Russian citizens as their natural destiny. Putin has woven the "chosen traumas" and the "chosen glories" of his country into an overarching "chosen myth" that transcends political ideology and offers a quasi-spiritual belief system founded on ideas of ethnic unity. Within this narrative, Ukraine is the culprit for wanting to be independent of Russia and

Russia is the aggrieved and innocent Motherland. The West is perceived as the historical enemy out to undermine and erode Russian culture and sovereignty. As this narrative unfolds, we can see that just as collective blame can be dangerous its partner, collective innocence, can also be deadly.

The central and underlying cause of blame is our experience of loss. In my concluding Epilogue, I reiterate that we blame others who hurt us through our wish for justice, as a means of rectifying the harm done, in our wish to return to a state of being intact, and, most importantly, to erase the scars that signify the loss we have suffered. Loss is the single most traumatic experience of our lives; it can either bring us together in our shared humanity or it can create lasting enmity and destruction. In the psychoanalytic process, healing comes about when the individual is able to accept his or her losses without being able to change what has happened or to change those who have inflicted harm. In the case of large groups and nations, the most important lesson we can learn, and perhaps the most difficult, is to find a way of accepting our loss without the hope of restitution.

Notes

1 Atrocity in this context means killing and/or maiming a targeted group of people in order to either exterminate them altogether, as in the case of genocide, or to subjugate them through cruel and inhumane treatment.
2 A version of Chapter Two has been published in *Psychoanalytic Perspectives on the Shadow of the Parent*, edited by J. Burke, Routledge, 2019. This chapter focuses on the children of perpetrators as carriers of collective guilt.

Chapter 1

Who's to Blame?

There has to be someone to blame. Otherwise, how would we make sense of things?
(John, divorced)

Introduction

This is a book about how we explain our history, both individually and collectively, how we resolve or fail to resolve conflict, how we perceive victims and perpetrators and how this can shift over time, and how we understand our role in shaping our lives, whether as agents or as subject to the whims of fate. These questions are also fundamental to the process of psychoanalysis whereby individuals who have been traumatized in their past seek a way of making sense of what has happened to them and how to break the spell of continuing to be victimized and continuing to place themselves in this position. In this process, the question of blame is central – who was the perpetrator, who caused the hurt, who is the one to blame?

Whenever misfortune occurs, we tend to blame someone even if there is no-one to blame. This gives us an illusion of power, that we are nevertheless in control, and allows us to direct our aggression at an imaginary culpable party. A tsunami may be attributed to the ire of the gods and even diseases such as COVID-19 are seen as someone's fault, in this case the Chinese. Trump notoriously blamed the raging forest fires in Oregon on mishandling by the state's Forestry Department. In reducing the unprecedented ferocity of the fires to human misconduct, Trump effectively denied any role that climate change might have played, reinstating the dearly held American illusion, going back to the early settlers' struggle for survival, that we are in control – or ought to be – of our environment. This form of irrational blame also, paradoxically, negates the possibility of real agency because it does not allow us to come to terms with what we cannot control. We resort to identifying a culprit as a way of understanding and accounting for a collective experience that has been chaotic and life-threatening. The more extreme the threat, the greater the need to apportion blame. Paradoxically, this defense only creates further insecurity because it undermines reality and the limits of our agency.

DOI: 10.4324/9781003379980-2

On an individual level, when we feel threatened blame can also be an effective form of abuse to control or gain power over someone else. A patient of mine explained why he avoided arguments with his wife. He said, "They turn into blaming matches. Either it's all my fault or I think it's all her fault. We reach a complete impasse very quickly and then there's no point in continuing. It usually ends up that I have to give in and do penance. But nothing is ever resolved." We've all experienced blaming matches at one time or another, or with one person or another, and know that, unless there was a genuine mistake that can be rectified, casting blame may seem the righteous thing to do but it may be destructive and misleading, imbuing a power balance in the relationship that often determines the dynamics of the relationship in the future. In the stalemate that ensues, both parties can continue to harbor resentment and hatred towards the other while denying their own aggression and destructiveness. It is a perfect sado-masochistic *folie à deux* in which self-harm, in the form of penance, is used passively to further harm the other. Guilt is passed back and forth like a hot potato and becomes the currency that keeps the relationship alive while each party masks their sadism in self-righteousness. This kind of sado-masochistic power battle is also evident in intransigent, longstanding political conflicts between groups or nations.

Our need to feel powerful is especially acute when we have been traumatized at the hands of others. The hallmark of patients who have been abused as children is that, although they see themselves as victims, they consciously blame themselves for their misfortunes – they were difficult or hateful children, faulty or demanding, and deserving ill treatment. By blaming themselves, they could maintain a good image of their parents and the world at large along with the belief that if only they could change themselves, "do penance", they could also be good – and loved. In later life these patients tend to blame authority figures or loved ones for the damage they suffer when unconsciously they are blaming the parents whom they still need to protect. This dynamic is also apparent in processes of reconciliation between antagonistic groups in which those identified as perpetrators are encouraged to apologize to their victims. False guilt, in the form of peace-making "penance", perpetuates the denial of real hatred and its causes and eventually re-surfaces in further acts of aggression. It is only when we can fully blame the objects of our anger and hurt, that we can begin to identify with them and accept our own capacity to make mistakes and to harm others.

While most of us as individuals develop a more nuanced and realistic view of blame through normal development or through the process of analysis, this is not so evident in the psychology of large group behavior, especially when longstanding conflicts define the relationship. Nothing is so frightening as being at the mercy of forces more powerful than us that do not conform to our social norms and rupture our worldview. On a collective level, as in the case of war, we need to know who our enemy is to defend ourselves and our collective actions. Notably it is always another country that either starts a war or provokes one's own country into aggression. In these cases, blame serves several purposes: it marks the enemy and in so doing strengthens group identity, it establishes the "rightness" of the social order that has been attacked, it justifies and absolves aggression towards the "other", and it creates a narrative of conflict that the group can adhere to and identify with.

Our initial reaction to loss or injury, of any kind, is to ask who or what is to blame? We want to find the culprit to set things right again, to restore justice and a world of moral order, and to transform the aggrieved from a helpless victim into a person with the power to seek retribution. Blame assumes a certain degree of agency on the part of the offender but it also confers a degree of power to the victim; in both positions blame assures us of some sense of control over our world – even if it is illusory at times.

The Purifying Scapegoat

At the heart of abuses of power and genocidal atrocities, minority groups are targeted to carry the blame for the social ills that beset the larger group. They also become the repository for all the shameful, primitive qualities attributed to being human, especially envy, greed and lawlessness. Moreover, when a large group's specific identity is at stake, a minority group is singled out as challenging, if not breaking the social order; order (and identity) can then only be restored through expulsion or, as René Girard, the historian and philosopher, argues, sacrifice. We see this across the world throughout history when the identity and survival of large groups is under threat. The large group typically reacts by means of self-purification and the demonization of "outsiders" who are depicted as the source of corruption and destruction of the group's sense of power as embodied in its identity. Identifying the minority group that poses the threat to the large group is the first step of differentiation, leading to expulsion if not outright extermination, whether it be the Jews in the case of Nazi Germany, the Tutsis in the case of Rwanda, the Mexicans in the case of Trump's populism, or the Uighurs in China. In each case, the malign intent of the group is unconsciously projected onto the demonized "other"; Hitler was particularly skilled at turning the group that was being victimized into the aggressor; for example, it was the Jews who were associated with Bolshevism, who were "subhuman" and a threat to German culture. Similarly, it was Poland that provoked German invasion in self-defense. More recently, in the wake of the Democrat victory in the Georgia elections, Trump accused the Democrats of "stealing" votes, an act which Trump might have hoped to achieve himself.[1] By accusing the Democrats of "stealing" votes, Trump was also consolidating his supporters in re-framing their defeat as an act of deliberate victimization, thereby justifying further attack and blame on the "other" who carries all the sins of the perpetrator.

Through this process of scapegoating, leading to ritualized if not actual murder, the group is politically cleansed, the social contract renewed, and identity re-established through the assertion of difference, demonstrating that the group possesses special powers and entitlement over others. Bringing about difference is essential to make the group superior, just as Britain and the United States claimed in their mirror mantras of "Make Britain/America Great Again!" This was also of course Hitler's promise to the defeated German nation. But in order for this process to be effective, the differentiation between good and bad needs to be clearly drawn so there is no moral or social ambiguity.

It is also essential that the group's goodness or sanctity is personified by a leader who represents the truth and who is beyond reproach. We have seen this in totalitarian leaders who resemble all-powerful emperors, close to God. Manning Clark, an Australian student based for a time at Bonn University, noted in his diary dated 11th December 1938, a month after Kristallnacht, a conversation with a retired professor of physics about the Jewish question. The professor, who was Jewish, could not accept that Hitler had anything to do with the violence against the Jews or indeed, if he had, would have allowed it to happen. Clark observed, "This was the first time I realized that the person of Hitler was sacrosanct. He was never connected in any way with instances that were doubtful or likely to prove unpopular. It was always Goring or Goebbels. Hitler's reputation is unblemished and for the normal German there is a halo of infallibility around his head" (Boyd, 2017, p.347). The retired professor and his family were subsequently sent to Theresienstadt concentration camp.

The sanctity of the leader preserves moral order within the group and establishes group cohesion, while blame for internal corruption or mistakes is located elsewhere. Scapegoats can always be found, either within or outside a nation. In the case of national emergencies, which are invariably prone to mishaps and mishandling, we see very plainly how leaders protect themselves. During the Chernobyl disaster, it was the firemen, the miners and the army who were deployed to put out the fire at the nuclear reactor; they became national heroes, sacrificing their lives for the safety of their country. Their sacrifice also significantly diverted attention away from the government leaders who had known about the weakness in the plant and had not done anything to rectify it. Sacrifice in this situation bolstered the Russian totalitarian ideology that emphasized the importance of the group over the individual. One Russian commentator explained:

> They were young lads. They're dying now too, but they know that, but for what they did … These are still people from a particular culture. A culture of superhuman feats and sacrificial victims … Our ideology? You are offered the choice of dying and acquiring meaning. They raise you up. They give you a role! It is worth dying because, afterwards, you will be immortal.
>
> (Alexievich, 2016, pp.173–4)

A Russian teacher also points to the ideal of struggle and sacrifice in the culture, saying,

> ... we have to go where it is difficult and dangerous and be ready to defend our Motherland. What else have I been teaching the children? Precisely that. You have to go into battle, rush into the line of fire, defend, sacrifice. The literature I was teaching was not about life: it was about war and death.
>
> (Ibid., p.180)

A culture of suffering gives meaning to the hardships of life (and those imposed by the political regime) and fosters a kind of blind faith in the leaders. Most importantly, the "mistakes" made in signing off the reactor as "safe" were rapidly removed from public scrutiny by re-framing the accident as a situation of warfare. As another Russian commented, "They call it 'an accident', 'a disaster', but it was a war. Our Chernobyl monuments resemble war memorials" (Ibid., p.177). In the aftermath of the Chernobyl meltdown, it was the scientists, not the politicians, who were ultimately held responsible and blamed. The politicians had won the war.

A similar process of diverting blame can be seen in the way in which the UK government has handled the COVID-19 pandemic.[2] Although the pandemic is a natural, not a manmade, disaster, the way in which leaders have tried to contain it and to minimize damage has varied considerably. While in the West we are aware of the Chinese early repression of news about the virus, it has taken some time to expose the fact that the British government failed to impose quarantine restrictions early enough and failed in their efforts to provide protective medical equipment early enough. Preferential contracts for medical equipment have also only recently been exposed. These failings have, however, been masked, similarly, in adopting a warfare mentality with special recognition given to the "heroes" of the National Health Service, especially those serving on the front lines. These "heroic" servants of the state, many of whom have lost their lives in the call of duty, are also the same servants, like the firemen and miners in Chernobyl, who have had to continue to do their jobs despite the incompetence and corruption of their leaders. But who can blame the leaders when a country is struggling to survive?

Arendt and the Concept of Collective Guilt

In the wake of atrocities, such as the Holocaust, blame is often targeted at the leader, ignoring the role of those followers who legitimize the leader's power. While it can be argued that leaders do have ultimate responsibility, this does not exculpate those who have followed orders. As leader of the Third Reich, Hitler held ultimate responsibility for the Final Solution, but what about all the other state officials and citizens who knowingly went along with this? And how are guilt and responsibility portioned out when large groups are involved?

On an individual basis, there is invariably a spectrum from agreement to compliance to resistance or defiance that comes into play in every situation and may also change over time within the individual. What someone believes is the right thing to do one day, may become the wrong thing on another day seen in a different light. In addition, different and often opposing sets of beliefs can co-exist within the same person. A simple and benign example is when people at a dinner party apparently agree with opinions that in private they would normally eschew. Techniques of denial and dissociation are commonly used to manage the cognitive dissonance between internal moral principles and external reality. In the case of perpetrators, the historian, Mary Fulbrook, describes what she refers to as "distancing", a form of dissociation:

> For those close to the atrocities, geographical distance was no excuse. Instead, many perpetrators adopted less literal forms of distance, detaching the self that acted in a particular situation from the "authentic" self and suggesting that the person who acted or behaved in certain ways was not the "real me". The "real" self is the moral inner self; the outwardly visible self that acted was prompted by external considerations over which it had little or no control. The easiest defense was to claim that they had merely followed orders in a situation where there had been no alternatives.
>
> (Fulbrook, 2018, p.417)

Of course, some perpetrators genuinely believe that atrocities in certain circumstances are justifiable, or that, in short, the ends justify the means and are not conflicted about what they have done. The natural comparison here is with the soldier who kills his enemy for the sake of winning the war. Although killing another human being is a difficult thing to do,[3] it can nevertheless be condoned within certain belief systems, such as self-defense, warfare, or the protection of others.

However, there are those perpetrators who experience moral conflict but who, as Fulbrook describes, find ways of continuing to comply with, if not actively support, a brutal regime.[4] In these cases it might be helpful to conceptualize a "functional" self that enables the individual to participate and belong to a group for the purpose of survival. This form of distancing or splitting may be a necessary technique for survival, but it falls apart when the question arises as to which self should or can be held responsible for an individual's actions. Which is the guilty self? Degrees of responsibility and guilt, particularly when the defense is that the accused was following orders, are some of the complexities that the Nuremberg Trials attempted to disentangle and remain to this day conceptually muddled and confusing.

Arendt was amongst the first writers and philosophers at that time to question collective morality and responsibility, propounding the view that, existentially, we are all to blame. This was also echoed by Primo Levi in his writing. If we accept this argument, does this mean we are all collectively guilty because we are all part of humanity? While most of us concur that, as social beings, we share certain responsibilities over our collective actions, our need to blame someone else and to exonerate ourselves remains a powerful political and social force that shapes our relations with other countries and within our own countries.

Since the Holocaust and atrocities committed in other parts of the world, moral pressure has been put on groups identified as perpetrators to admit to their crimes and, in doing so, to perform an act of social cleansing. This dynamic has recently surfaced in the far left in the US as white people are held accountable for the sins of their slaveholding forebears. As members of a group, we may all be responsible for the well-being and behavior of the group but this does not necessarily mean that if one of its members commits a crime we are all guilty. Nor does it mean that the group is guilty for its crimes in the past. We abhor, for example, the idea that the children of a murderer will be consequently stigmatized as untrustworthy or even dangerous. There is a difference between the concept of collective guilt and collective responsibility that is of paramount importance to our current debate about collective guilt. This difference crucially shifts the balance from blame to the recognition of social responsibility, to our social contract in the present and going forward to the future.

Arendt criticizes the concept of collective guilt for a number of reasons, but above all she emphasizes the importance of distinguishing it from the idea of collective responsibility. In her essay, "Collective Responsibility", she writes:

> There is such a thing as responsibility for things one has not done; one can be held liable for them. But there is no such thing as being or feeling guilty for things that happened without oneself actively participating in them. This is an important point, worth making loudly and clearly at a moment when so many good white liberals confess to guilt feelings with respect to the Negro question. I do not know how many precedents there are in history for such misplaced feelings, but I do know that in post-war Germany, where similar problems arose with respect to what had been done by the Hitler regime to the Jews, the cry "We are all guilty" that at first hearing sounded so very noble and tempting has actually only served to exculpate to a considerable degree those who actually were guilty. Where all are guilty, nobody is. Guilt, unlike responsibility, always singles out; it is strictly personal. It refers to an act, not to intentions or potentialities. It is only in a metaphorical sense that we can say we *feel* guilty for the sins of our fathers or our people or mankind, in short, for deeds we have not done, although the course of events may well make us pay for them.
>
> (Arendt, 2003, p.147)

This essay was written in 1968. In making the distinction between "feeling" guilty and being guilty, Arendt is pointing out what we can describe as a neurotic form of collective guilt. She goes on to make the point that for such emotions as collective guilt, "solidarity is a necessary condition" and explains, "in our case of collective guilt feelings would mean that the cry 'We are all guilty' is actually a declaration of solidarity with the wrongdoers" (Ibid., p.148). This analysis of collective solidarity is evident in the psychoanalytic context in the common tendency of patients to protect their parents by taking on their sins and in this way exculpating them. Through this neurotic form of identification, as Arendt claims, everyone is guilty and no one is. The parents (or in the case of large groups, the authorities) on which the children rely are not held solely responsible for their misdeeds because this would necessitate separation from them and condemnation. The family or group is held together through guilt. This is different, however, from sharing collective responsibility.

The essential difference that Arendt wants us to acknowledge has to do with the role of the individual within the political realm. She emphasizes that it is only the individual who can be guilty of crimes, not the collective, as it is only the individual who is able to think and act with agency. She explains:

> Whether the defendant was a member of the Mafia or a member of the SS or some other criminal or political organization, assuring us that he was a mere cog who acted only upon superior orders and did what everybody else would have done just as well, the moment he appears in a court of justice he appears as a person and is judged according to what he did. It is the grandeur of court proceedings that even a cog can become a person again.
>
> (Ibid., p.148)

By placing guilt at the feet of the individual, Arendt is restoring our capacity to think and to make judgments as human beings. This is antithetical to a totalitarian framework in which the individual is a "cog" within the larger group and it is the group's survival, no matter the means, that is paramount. To hold the group guilty of wrongdoing not only absolves its members of having any individual agency or authority but it also confirms the totalitarian nature of the group.

Collective responsibility, Arendt goes on to argue, must meet two conditions:

> I must be held responsible for something I have not done, and the reason for my responsibility must be my membership in a group (a collective) which no voluntary act of mine can dissolve ... This kind of responsibility in my opinion is always political, whether it appears in the older form, when a whole community takes it upon itself to be responsible for whatever one of its members has done, or whether a community is being held responsible for what has been done in its name ... Every government

assumes responsibility for the deeds and misdeeds of its predecessors and every nation for the deeds and misdeeds of the past.

(Ibid., p.149)

Although Arendt specifies that this kind of responsibility "is always political", this is a bit like saying every group can be qualified as political. Within the family group, for example, mutual ties and dependency create mutual responsibility by virtue of being a member of the family, but this is not the same thing as implying that every member of the family is guilty of the misdeeds of one of its members. As Arendt states,

no moral, individual and personal, standards of conduct will ever be able to excuse us from collective responsibility. This vicarious responsibility for things we have not done, this taking upon ourselves the consequences for things we are entirely innocent of, is the price we pay for the fact that we live our lives not by ourselves but among our fellow men, and that the faculty of action, which, after all, is the political faculty par excellence, can be actualized only in one of the many and manifold forms of human community.

(Ibid., pp.157–8)

Because we live as humans within collective societies, we are necessarily responsible for what we create and for our collective actions. An integral part of our collective responsibility is to hold the individual to account for his/her deeds that affect others. While Germany, for example, as a nation is responsible for its past and its present, including acknowledgment of wrongdoing, it is nevertheless individual citizens who must be held to account. This does not mean that those who did not resist the Reich did not experience conflicts of conscience or feel tainted by the crimes committed that were more commonly known than we had imagined. This crosses into the territory of sins of omission. But neither is it right to confer guilt onto those who have not engaged in criminality for the actions of others who have.

Perverse Cycles of Blame

Returning to my example of the couple who continually blame one another for their conflicts, we can see how blame can be used to maintain the conflict and not to resolve it, or, if it is unresolvable, not to accept this either. This is apparent in long-standing intransigent conflicts between nations and ethnic groups in which the conflict has taken the form of a grudge or endless vendetta that has become an integral aspect of group identity, marking difference between the warring parties. Freud's concept of the narcissism of minor differences enables us to understand how demonizing the "other" functions as a way of maintaining stability and a sense of group identity, especially, and paradoxically, when there is no common external enemy and relative security within the group. At times of peace, for example, internal conflicts within a group can come to the surface and threaten to fragment the group.

While Freud roots his idea of the narcissism of minor difference in the narcissistic threat presented by sexual difference, Girard views the basis for envy and violence in what he refers to as human "mimetic desire", i.e. that it is our innate proclivity to imitate each other and hence to desire what they deem desirable, that creates envy and competition to the point of violence. When groups are not struggling to maintain their borders against the enemy, the struggle for what may be an illusory possession of what is seen to be desirable occurs internally. Having experienced decades of relative peace and prosperity, we have witnessed in the last ten years or so increasing political conflict and divisions within both the European Union and the United States.

This leads us to the question of peace and war and how they interplay with the identity of large groups. There is a strong argument, supported by sociologists such as Max Weber and Georg Simmel, and political scientists such as Michael Desch, that war is the most important factor in establishing "strong, centralized states and cohesive national polities" (Walt, 2016). The impetus to fight the enemy requires internal unity while it also promotes patriotism and the suppression of internal divisions. But as Simmel points out: "A group's complete victory over its enemies is … not always fortunate … Victory lowers the energy which guarantees the unity of the group; and the dissolving forces, which are always at work, gain hold" (Ibid.).

There are numerous examples of the drawbacks to victory and peace throughout history. Here are two brief examples. In Europe, the period from 1815 and the Treaty of Paris until the Crimean War of 1853 was relatively free from external threats. Yet during this same period there was an unprecedented breakdown in state cohesion and a series of internal upheavals across various European states. In the US, by 1850 external threats were inconsequential and yet by 1860 the American Civil War was about to erupt.

In contrast, the Cold War gave birth to the American federal state and strengthened national unity. Desch describes the Cold War as the "perfect type of threat" (Ibid.). It did not escalate to a state of war but it served to unify the states under threat and to enhance their alliance with one another. Since the end of the Cold War, the level of conflict in the world has generally been declining. While there is greater stability, this also allows internal conflicts to surface and become more divisive.[5] Desch argues, "The longer the period of reduced international security competition, the more likely are developed states to be plagued by the rise of narrow sectoral, rather than broad encompassing, interest groups" (Ibid.).

The lesson here is that reducing external dangers has a downside. Stephen Walt, Professor of International Relations at Harvard, argues: "The less threatened we are by the outside world, the more prone we are to ugly quarrels at home. Even worse, peace may contain the seeds of its own destruction.

As we are now seeing in the Middle East, the collapse of unity and state authority can easily trigger violent internal conflicts that eventually drag outside powers back in" (Ibid.).

Girard makes two important observations about cycles of violence and blame within societies. The first and, according to Robert Pogue Harrison, most valuable insight,

> is that rivalry and violence arise from sameness rather than difference. Where conflicts erupt between neighbors or ethnic groups, or even among nations, more often than not it's because of what they have in common rather than what distinguishes them. In Girard's words: "The error is always to reason within categories of 'difference' when the root of all conflicts is rather 'competition,' mimetic rivalry between persons, countries, cultures."
>
> (Harrison, 2018)

Often we fight or go to war to prove our difference from an enemy who in fact resembles us in ways we are all too eager to deny.[6]

A related insight of equal importance concerns the deadly cycles of revenge and reciprocal violence. The declared wish to restore justice may also cloak the desire for revenge, to inflict even greater violence. Girard taught that retaliation hardly ever limits itself to "an eye for an eye" but almost always escalates the level of violence. Every escalation is imitated in turn by the other party:

> Clausewitz sees very clearly that *modern wars are as violent as they are only because they are "reciprocal"*: mobilization involves more and more people until it is "total," as Ernst Junger wrote of the 1914 war ... It was because he was "responding" to the humiliations inflicted by the Treaty of Versailles and the occupation of the Rhineland that Hitler was able to mobilize a whole people. Likewise, it was because he was "responding" to the German invasion that Stalin achieved a decisive victory over Hitler. It was because he was "responding" to the United States that Bin Laden planned 9/11 ... The one who believes he can control violence by setting up defenses is in fact controlled by violence. These remarks come from the last book Girard wrote, *Battling to the End* (2010).
>
> (Harrison, 2018)

In this book, Girard discusses with Benoît Chantre, the French Girardian, war theorist Carl von Clausewitz's ideas about the "escalation of violence" in modern warfare which closely accord with Girard's ideas about the acceleration of mimetic violence. In the example of the endless accusations and counter-accusations between my patient and his wife, we can see this escalating dynamic of blame that ultimately leads to the destruction of a cooperative relationship and spawns a perverse relationship based on hatred. Girard points out that the word "Satan" in Hebrew means "accuser" or "adversary" and warns us against the perverse, satanic element of the impassioned accuser that can lead to a dangerous confusion between guilt and innocence.

Beyond Blame

Ultimately, as Girard argues, it is only the scapegoat who can accept blame and embody the sins of the community. The Biblical ritual of the scapegoat vividly illustrates this process: one kid goat is sacrificed to appease God while the other living kid goat is expelled into the wilderness, carrying away the iniquities of the community "to a barren region" (Leviticus 16:21–22). The act of sacrifice and expulsion breaks, or is intended to break, the escalation of violence. It has the power to do this not because it is an act of atonement but because it signifies an act of acknowledgment – the acknowledgment of human destructiveness, of original sin. In this respect, it is perhaps close to what Arendt describes as collective responsibility insofar as we are born with original sin.

In the novel, *We Germans*, the narrator, a former German soldier serving under the Reich, captures the ambiguous convergence of guilt and responsibility,

> When I ask myself whether we were all immoral, or whether having done wrong makes us evil men, I think that we were blemished by the consequences of what other people decided. No one ever has complete responsibility for his own moral balance. And the unforgiving truth, the severe, ancient truth, is that you can be culpable for something that you weren't in control of.
>
> (Starritt, 2020, Loc.332)

Conferring guilt onto a group for misdeeds committed under its name in the past is not only fraught with the problem of collapsing different categories of guilt and responsibility into one undifferentiated mass but it can also, paradoxically, detract from our collective responsibility going forwards into the future. It is easy enough, for example, to say, "How could the Germans have committed such inhuman crimes?" with the insinuation that it is only the Germans who could do such a thing, not those of us who are not German. The use of guilt in this context not only further demonizes the "other" while it purifies "us", but in doing so there is no recognition that we must, as collective societies, all take responsibility so that this doesn't happen on our watch. The political scientist, Iris Marion Young, makes an important distinction about collective responsibility:

> The meaning of political responsibility is forward-looking. One *has* the responsibility always *now*, in relation to current events and in relation to their future consequences. We are in a condition of having such political

responsibility, and the fact of having it implies an imperative to *take* political responsibility … In this sense political responsibility is forward-looking: it means in the first stance taking up a responsibility to be political.

(Young, 2011, p.92)

Notes

1 In a phone call on 2nd January 2021, prior to the state elections, Trump demanded that Brad Raffensperger, Georgia's Secretary of State and a Republican, "find" him enough votes to overturn his election defeat. Raffensperger refused.
2 This is not to suggest that there has been no corruption or mishandling of the pandemic in other countries across the world, but in 2022 the UK had the highest per capita mortality rate of the virus in Western Europe. This reflects differences in policies and government actions; it is not due to difference in the virus.
3 See Collins, R. (2008), *Violence: A Micro-sociological Theory*. Princeton: Princeton University Press.
4 For a full discussion of the psychology of perpetrators, see Chapter 2, "Hannah Arendt and the Eradication of Thought" in Covington, C. (2017). *Everyday Evils: A Psychoanalytic View of Evil and Morality*. London: Routledge.
5 Russia's invasion of Ukraine on 24th February 2022 marked a turning point in the tide of international conflict, creating a shift in the consolidation of Western alliances with the resurgence of Cold War tensions.
6 Girard's argument that we go to war "to prove our difference from an enemy" is especially apposite in relation to the UK's recent separation from the EU. The practical ramifications, at least in economic terms, are generally considered detrimental to the UK. It is estimated that there will be a drop of 2.1% in the national GDP compared to if Britain had remained within the EU. Politically, however, the Leave campaign has notably stressed sovereignty and "Taking Back Control" as its aim, indicating that a central problem may have been precisely what Girard points to – that the UK no longer felt different enough from other EU countries and therefore distinct in its power.

References

Alexievich, S. (2016). *Chernobyl Prayer*. London: Penguin Books.

Arendt, H. (2003). *Responsibility and Judgment*. New York: Schocken Books.

Boyd, J. (2017). *Travellers in the Third Reich*. London: Elliott & Thompson Ltd.

Fulbrook, M. (2018). *Reckonings: Legacies of Nazi Persecution and the Quest for Justice*. Oxford: Oxford University Press.

Harrison, R.P. (20 December 2018). "The Prophet of Envy." *New York Review of Books*.

Leviticus 16. *Bible*. New Revised Standard Version.

Starritt, A. (2020). *We Germans*. London: John Murray.

Walt, S.M. (17 June 2016). "The Case Against Peace." *Foreign Policy*.

Young, I.M. (2011). *Responsibility for Justice*. Oxford: Oxford University Press.

Chapter 2

A Tragic Inheritance

The Irresolvable Conflict for Children of Perpetrators[1]

> I can't help what my parents did, or my grandparents, but does that mean I
> have to feel guilty for the horrors they committed?
>
> (Karin, German SS family)

Introduction

In her reflections on the aftermath of the German Reich, Eva Hoffman
describes the experience of children of survivors of the *Shoah* (the Holocaust).
She writes:

> ... what we children received, with great directness, were the emotional
> sequelae of our elders' experiences, the acid-etched traces of what they
> had endured. This perhaps, is always the way in which one generation's
> legacy is actually passed on to the next – through the imprint of personal
> and historical experiences as these are traced on individual psyches and
> sensibilities. But ... the traces left on the survivors' psyches were not so
> much thoughts or images as scars and wounds. The legacy they passed on
> was not a processed, mastered past, but the splintered signs of acute
> suffering, of grief and loss.
>
> (Hoffman, 2004, p.34)

Efraim Sicher refers to the invisible scars of the next generation, "the scar
without the wound", as the marks of trauma, experienced not in real time but
in a timeless psychic reality, affecting identity and the sense of self in relation
to the world (Sicher, 1998, p.27). Hoffman clearly states, "For me, in the
beginning was the war, and the Holocaust was the ontological basis of my
universe" (Hoffman, p.278). The trauma of the parents, both individually and
in this case as a group, resides in the unconscious of their children, silently
shaping their internal world and their actions in the external world.

There is now an extensive literature on the transgenerational effects of
trauma, and of Holocaust survivors in particular.[2] Starting in the late 1980s,

DOI: 10.4324/9781003379980-3

a body of literature and film emerged giving recognition to the children of Nazi perpetrators and highlighting their own difficulties in coming to terms with the past of their parents.[3] Comparisons between the two groups are inevitable but also fraught with conceptual and experiential contradictions and problems. I will touch on some of these similarities and differences later in this chapter. However, there is a principal distinction between these groups, articulated by Dan Bar-On in *The Indescribable and the Undiscussable* (Bar-On, 1999). Bar-On distinguishes between a trauma that is too painful to talk about and a history that cannot be talked about, that has been "effaced from normalized discourse" (McGlothlin, 2006, p.6, footnote). Hoffman argues that the latter cannot be classed as a trauma, with the implication of victimization, but as a tragedy. She explains, "For tragedy, of course, involves a conflict – agon – between opposing principles and agents. Trauma is produced by persecution of subjects to whom all agency and principle have been denied" (Hoffman, p.41). Perpetrators, on the other hand, have acted out a tragic conflict that then casts a shadow over their offspring and generations to come. The discovery that one's parents have committed evil acts throws up fundamental conflicts that affect the child's identity, sense of morality, and worldview.

In this chapter, I will present clinical material from work with a young woman whose father had been a leading military figure in a bloody civil war and had ultimately been indicted for torture. Her material touches on many aspects of the experiences of children of Nazi perpetrators. While the relationship of each child with his/her parent necessarily varies, taken together these stories form a composite that sheds light on children of perpetrators in other similar situations, e.g. of the genocides in Cambodia, Rwanda, Kosovo, Syria, and so on. It is important to clarify that these are perpetrators who have been involved in what would qualify as *evil acts that have been sanctioned by a higher authority*. I am defining evil in this context as an act intended to dehumanize another group of people who are distinctly targeted and categorized by race, religion, political affiliation, or place, to the point of extermination.

While there are numerous examples of children of criminally violent parents who also struggle with the contamination and shame this incurs on the family,[4] this is an intrinsically different experience to that of a child whose parent has perpetrated atrocities that are sanctioned by society. I also make the distinction between children of parents who have participated in extreme violence in armed conflict that is sanctioned and is not deemed evil. In these cases, while the parent's experiences may have been traumatic, the parent is generally perceived as a hero or fighting for a heroic cause, not as a demon who is corrupted by evil.

Case Study: Living in the Cracks

Ana contacted me on the advice of her doctor because of recurring severe headaches that she had experienced over the last two years since her recent marriage. She also mentioned that she had nightmares of being attacked that made her feel very anxious.

Ana appeared for our first meeting exactly on time, immediately removed her shoes and left them by the front door, and hung up her coat on the hook I indicated. She was a very attractive woman, conservatively well dressed, and smiled at me as if she was inviting me to speak. This left a strange sensation in me of not just a reversal of roles but of being kept out by her, despite her seeming warmth. There was a brief silence and she then told me that at the age of 15 she and her mother, her younger brother and her baby sister had emigrated from their country of origin in the aftermath of terrible civil war. She told me in great detail about their harrowing escape, catching lifts from trucks, hiding in goods train carriages, and walking along deserted mountain paths with nothing to eat and no shelter. She smiled and said she had kept a diary of this time and was going to write a book about it someday.

Although her story was remarkable and she could express how very frightening is was at times, I was struck by the fact that it didn't seem to be the problem. Not knowing what to say, I asked her whether she thought there was some link between her headaches and her nightmares and this traumatic period in her life. Ana looked at me and said,

> No, I don't think there is a link because that's over now. It was a terrible time but it was also full of the excitement of a new life and freedom from what had happened in our country. My headaches only started when I got married and this is what I can't understand. I love my husband and he is very kind and loving to me. He is everything I could wish for, but I'm afraid I will somehow ruin everything.

Ana had eagerly agreed to see me three times a week and voluntarily asked if she could lie on my couch, not facing me. During the first few weeks, she dutifully arrived on time, lay on the couch and embellished her stories about her family's great escape, as if hoping we would find some clue from them to alleviate her headaches. She also picked her way through her feelings towards her husband, but there again it was clear she loved him and they had a good marriage. Then silence. I was beginning to feel a mixture of despair and doubt as to whether in fact Ana's headaches were analyzable and I had made a mistake in taking her on as a patient.

In the following session, as Ana was recounting another episode in her escape saga, she remembered a dream from the previous night. In her dream she was seeing a doctor or perhaps it was a friend, she wasn't sure, who was going to give her some medicine for her headaches. Ana was wearing long white delicate kid gloves and the doctor asked her to remove them. She removed her right-hand glove but then hesitated with her left hand. The doctor insisted it was necessary to remove both and Ana reluctantly took off the glove from her left hand, revealing that her left hand had become disfigured as the muscles had atrophied. Ana was shocked to see what had happened but, more than this, she felt deeply ashamed to show the doctor something so grotesque in her.

I asked Ana what she thought of the dream and, after a moment, she replied that her father was left-handed and the family had always teased him about this. It made her wonder whether she was in some way like him.

Ana's response made me realize that she had never mentioned her father and that I too had blanked him out, as if he had not existed. I said, "I'm aware that in all your stories about the escape, you haven't mentioned your father once. Was he alive and, if so, where was he?"

Ana remained still for some time and simply said, "He stayed behind."

"Stayed behind?" I asked.

For the first time, Ana became irritated and answered sharply, "Yes! He stayed behind. Didn't you hear me?"

There was a long silence and Ana then relented,

> I'm sorry to be so rude. My father stayed behind because he was in prison. He's still in prison ... He's well known at home and after the war he was tried for torturing prisoners. He was found guilty. It's all out now, everyone knows. We couldn't stay after that. As soon as he was found guilty we started getting death threats. Everyone knew we were his family and in their eyes we were all to blame. He wrecked our lives there.

Ana's disclosure turned out to be the missing piece of the puzzle that enabled her to tell me about the events that had torn her family apart.

Like many children of Nazi perpetrators, Ana had described a very happy childhood and loving parents. Her father put his family first, providing well for them, ensuring they had the best of everything, and, although he was strict with the children, he was also gentle and loving. One example Ana gave of her father's kindness was when he caught her as a young child prodding a bird with a broken wing. She remembered him lecturing her about how cruel it was to torture animals and feeling ashamed and exposed before him. She commented, "This is not the same man who was found guilty of torture – how could he be the same?"

Ana was her father's favorite and had felt particularly close to him as a child, playing games and making up stories that were special between them. She remembered during the war an occasion when her mother had interrupted her from asking her father to play, explaining he was tired and needed to rest. Ana had felt irritated with her mother, whom she normally got along well with, and linked this to her irritation with me for asking her about where her father was. She said,

> I think it was the first time I became at all aware that there was something wrong. It wasn't that my father was tired, he looked ill, like he was

breaking apart and I didn't know what was going on. I was irritated that there was something I didn't know about and it was clear then that my parents knew. My parents never talked about what was going on outside our family and I had grown up thinking this was normal. My mother still doesn't. Of course, I knew that terrible things were happening in the war and my father was brave, but this was a different feeling. My father prided himself on being in control at all times – and this time he was cracking. It wasn't exactly a sadness that was the problem, it was something else indefinable. I remember when I was upset and cried when I was little and he didn't comfort me but he would say in a gentle voice, "You mustn't cry. It's important to be brave and strong and then you won't feel sad anymore." So I knew what it was like to be strong and not to be sad. I knew the war was going badly and we were losing and wondered if my father felt he had failed. It was so important for him to do his best and to do what was right.

Over the next few sessions, Ana told me about her father's trial, or what she knew of it, and described some of the allegations that had been made against her father. He was a high-ranking officer and had not only instigated the torture of prisoners but had also authorized localized mass killings. The evidence was clear that he had both given orders and had been directly involved in these events. His defense was consistently that he was doing his duty for his country, that the torture was required to obtain information and that the killings were for self-protection, particularly when his military unit was threatened with reprisals.

Ana admitted that, putting herself inside his mind, she could understand it all made sense. But when she looked at it from her perspective, she was horrified not only at what her father had done and had been capable of doing but of what she felt was a total betrayal of her. She suddenly complained of a headache coming on and started crying. She sobbed,

> This is so hard to live with. He is the father I have loved so much, who made me feel so loved, and he is now the father whom I hate for what he has done. How can I have any respect for him? Yet I still love him. This is why my head is splitting. I can't keep these two fathers together. And I don't know where this puts me.

An integral part of our childhood psychic development is the painful realization of hating the object of our love. However, for Ana, as for other children of perpetrators, the problem is not simply that of holding these opposites together. The problem is how to think about a father who has acted like a loving parent in one world and a monster in another. Ana was articulating how hard this is to live with – and to recognize – and what it means about her as a person and whether she could trust what she saw of herself in the mirror, as her view of her father and his reflection of her had cracked. At the same time she desperately wanted to protect the father of her childhood and deny he was responsible for the crimes he had committed.

In the sessions following Ana's insight about her splitting headaches, she became noticeably paranoid in her behavior towards me, accusing me of being critical of her, not believing her, and of pretending to be concerned about her. In the transference I alternated between being a father whom she could no longer trust and being her critical superego that castigated her for her hatred and sense of betrayal of her father. Ana began to see what she was projecting on to me and at the end of a session in which she had been especially rejecting of anything I said, she exclaimed,

> I don't want to be like this! But I'm also angry with you because I don't want to have to understand! I have to make someone – whether it's you or myself – an enemy. I don't know how else to manage what I know. I fluctuate from not wanting to believe any of it – that my father was really only my father and never did any of the horrible things he did – and from attacking myself for being so stupid not to have seen this before and wanting to kill him and everything about my past. I want to believe I've been duped all along – but then I remember other things … I can't find a place for what has happened inside me. I am left with this crap, this horrible hand in my dream that I can't get rid of. And I can't get rid of feeling I am to blame, I'm guilty!

Ana was trying to grasp the world that had been kept secret from her and to square this with her own experience. She spent hours venting her fury against her father, continually questioning how he could have done these things. Her anger and disbelief eventually gave way to trying to think about how her father had been able to justify what he was doing – how he could remain the same person. She saw his obsession with duty and doing his best as something which had resulted paradoxically in two very different outcomes. He was the dutiful father and the dutiful military leader – but what was admirable behavior in one context did not necessarily apply to another. Seeing how driven her father had been to perform well, Ana then remembered the time when she thought he was breaking apart. As if speaking to him, she said,

> I think that was the moment when you couldn't go on any longer, when you saw that all your efforts to do well, to be a good soldier, to be brave, to be loyal, all of it had failed and that was your tragedy and it's mine now. You believed what you were doing was for the right and then you were let down, it all crumbled and everyone could see the cracks. And now it's the cracks that I have to live in. You've covered them over and go on trying to convince yourself – but you can't be with me in my world any longer.

In finding some explanatory thread to keep her father's identity together, Ana was able to incorporate a fuller and more complex picture of him, and eventually of herself. She was not so naïve as to think that her father's fault line had been his propensity to follow orders, but this was the beginning of her understanding of how he could be the "same" person and how elusive the boundary between these seemingly different persons can be.

Ana's headaches stopped. She had reached some form of reconciliation with her father, accepting her love for him but at the same time knowing she could not be in contact with him because to do so would be to perpetuate the deceit between them. There was nothing she could say to him that could resolve this conflict.

She was nevertheless left with the question as to why her headaches had started soon after her marriage, especially as there seemed to be no significant problems in her marital life. Her persecutory dreams continued periodically and also signaled that she had her own internal demons to deal with. The penny dropped one afternoon when Ana heard herself talking about trying to be a dutiful wife. She turned round to face me as if wanting to confirm that I was there with her but, most importantly, that I was separate from her. She lay back again and said,

> That's it! You remember when I said I was worried I might do something to ruin my marriage? I have this dutiful streak in me just like my father – this flaw that can ruin everything if I'm not careful and if I let it rule me. I think all along I've known I have this and I've also sensed some danger inside me but I haven't been able to see what it was. I think it's what makes me feel so frightened in my dreams. I can also see that if I had been in my father's position, it is possible I could have behaved as he did. I hope I wouldn't have. But I can see how close this is inside me.

I commented that there might be another problem in trying so hard to be the dutiful wife as it might mean leaving things unspoken with her husband and jeopardizing their intimacy, as her father had done with his family. Her splitting headaches had contained the lacuna of what could not be spoken about, of a discrepancy she could not make sense of and yet could not suppress altogether.

Ana replied,

> It's true, I'm always watching myself, censoring what I say, as if some awful secret will come out. I put up a wall with my husband – and within myself.

Ana's awareness of her own proclivity to step over the boundary and enter into a perverse, dehumanizing world did not resolve the pain and betrayal she felt from her father and the rupture this had made in her life, but it did help her to bear the contamination her father had brought on the family and to become her own agent who could make different choices. It also enabled her to dismantle an internal wall she had constructed to keep what was so horrifying apart – in a hidden place inside her.

A Background of Silence

In listening to and reading accounts of the children of Nazi perpetrators, the most striking feature that stands out in their experience of family life is the silence surrounding what was going on in the outside world and, specifically, their fathers' involvement in these events that were unspeakable within the privacy of the family.[5] This was reflected in Ana's initial silence about her father and what I later realized was my unconscious collusion with this. Outside the confines of my consulting room, there was another reality that could not be spoken or thought about without serious breach of the world Ana had tried to preserve for herself and those close to her.

In some families there was a clear process of splitting whereby internal family life was idealized and revered, and the external world presented a struggle to contain and combat what was impure and life-threatening. Rudolf Hoess's daughter, Ingebirgitt, describes this split graphically in her memories of "my beautiful Auschwitz childhood" (Hall, 2015), living in ease in a house adjoining the perimeter of the concentration camp her father had designed and built. What happened on the other side of the garden wall was not known or spoken about. Despite the fact that the servants were often prisoners from the camp, the family maintained a wall of silence that was critical in maintaining the existence of these two seemingly antithetical worlds. Just as the garden wall physically demarcated a world of love from a world of hate, so did the silence.

While in retrospect we may want to interpret the silence experienced during the war as a form of denial or dissociation, it is important to acknowledge that for many families, such as Ana's, there was no conscious awareness of violations taking place. The belief system that enables atrocities to take place rests on adherence to duty and duty to a higher authority that is perceived to be safeguarding and promoting the interests of the group. In order to exist within this environment, especially when active engagement is required, the belief system needs to be upheld. Silence then serves to protect the group not only from the horrors of war but it suppresses questioning of the prevalent belief system. When atrocities do come to light at the end of a war, the ensuing shame and guilt are so intense that the need for silence then becomes acute – but it is a silence of a different order. In her War Diary, Ingeborg Bachmann writes about the impossibility of betraying her family "with its festering boils", explaining, "I have acquired a big eye for my family, a big ear for its languages, acquired a big silence about so much that is to be hushed up from the immediate proximity" (Bachmann, 2018, p.77). This was the silence that permeated Ana's family after leaving their homeland and a father imprisoned for war crimes.

Postwar silence within families could also be tinged with coldness and emotional distance. Hoffman describes children of perpetrators "growing up in homes where a heavy atmosphere of secrecy reigned; of parents perceived as chilly and distant; of subjects that were seen as untouchable, and of gradual or sudden realizations that something had been recently and deeply rotten in the state in which the children were growing up" (Hoffman, p.120). For a child, the presence of a secret held by the parents has profound emotional consequences, to the point where the child is unsure what to believe and what not to believe within the family history. There is also an inevitable sense of exclusion that casts a shadow over the child's sense of himself, conferring unconscious guilt as to whether the child himself has been the cause of something so terrible it cannot be spoken about. A borderline patient of mine, who grew up in a family involved with the French resistance, described a childhood of mysterious references to relatives who had disappeared and the fear it instilled in her and her siblings that this could either happen to them or that they would discover the truth and be murdered themselves. What she came to realize in the course of her analysis was that the threat of murder was her anxiety that unravelling the family history would destroy not only the fiction that the family had lived by but her own make-believe version of her parents and siblings.

The silent shrouding of the past is painfully portrayed in Bernhard Schlink's story about a son trying to make contact with his aging father. Schlink writes:

> Why did his questions pressure his father? Because he didn't want to turn his insides out, particularly in front of his son? Because his insides, where the doors and windows had never been opened, were all shrivelled and dead, and he didn't know what his son wanted of him? Because he's grown up before psychoanalysis and psychotherapy had made revelations a daily occurrence and he had no language to communicate his inner feelings? Because whatever he'd done and whatever happened to him, from his two marriages to his professional obligations before and after 1945, he saw in it such a continuity that it was in fact the same and there was nothing to say about it? ... Wordless intimacy had been too much to hope for.
>
> (Schlink, 2012, p.187)

Schlink's narrator struggles to understand his father's silence and in the end wonders whether it reveals what he describes as a "continuity", as if the silence itself maintains a connection between past and present that would be betrayed or broken by speech. There is then "nothing to say". This passage evokes what Hoffman refers to as a kind of "endorsed amnesia" during the postwar years in Germany, in which the subject of the Holocaust was virtually censored (Hoffman, p.120). She goes on to observe that when the postwar generation discovered the truth, it came as a shock and led to explosions within families and within German society, as if waking up *into* a nightmare. While Hoffman suggests that there was some form of mass repression, Schlink's question about "continuity" reveals the essential importance of maintaining an identity and set of beliefs underlying one's identity that continues over time, despite ruptures in one's experience of the world and oneself.

Repudiation, Idealization and Acceptance

My brief account of Ana's analysis illustrates only some of the features and conflicts experienced by children of perpetrators. Ana is also perhaps an exception because she sought an analysis to help her come to terms with her past. Overall, children of perpetrators seem to fall into three categories in terms of their relationships with their fathers; these categories can be broadly classed as idealization, repudiation and acceptance. Philippe Sands's film, *My Nazi Legacy*, vividly portrays the opposing relationships between two sons and their respective high-ranking Nazi fathers: Hans Frank, governor of occupied Poland and Otto von Wachter, governor of Galicia in Ukraine. Niklas Frank bitterly repudiates his father, Hans Frank, in contrast to Horst von Wachter, who idealizes his father, Otto von Wachter, refusing to accept the crimes he committed. But the distinctive difference between these men is that Niklas had a cold, unloving father whereas Horst viewed his father as "a good man, a liberal who did his best ... Others would have been worse" (Sands, 2016, p.246). For Niklas, the decisive moment in his relationship with his father is when, at the age of seven, he visits him in prison at the time of the Nuremberg Trials. Niklas remembers,

> I didn't say goodbye. The whole thing lasted not more than six or seven minutes. There were no tears. I was really sad. Sad that he lied to me. Sad that he didn't tell me the truth about what might happen to him. Sad about what would happen to us.
>
> (Sands, p.364)

This final estrangement and deceit contributed to Niklas's decision to repudiate his father, a repudiation made easy as it was consistent with his experience of his father.

For Horst, however, his loyalty to his father is a stumbling block that prevents him from repudiating his father and leaves him with a conflict. In Horst's attempt to preserve the good in his father, he transforms the narrative of his father from perpetrator to victim. He admits,

> I cannot say I love my father. I love my grandfather ... I have a responsibility for my father in some way, to see what really happened, to tell the

truth, and to do what I can do for him ... I have to find some positive aspect ... I know that the whole system was criminal and that he was part of it, but I don't think he was a criminal. He didn't act like a criminal ... There was no chance to leave the system ... he was completely in the system.

(Sands, pp.250–1)

As Sands observes, Horst was "on a mission of rehabilitation" (Sands, p.246). The problem with Horst's "rehabilitation" is that it is predicated on his father's innocence. What Horst cannot accept is that his father may have been a "good" man *and* he committed evil acts. This is the fundamental paradox that evil poses, particularly when evil acts occur *en masse*; that all evil deeds are committed by humans who also, by and large, have loving relationships.

Idealization effectively collapses the conflicting reality of the past but is at the cost of denying reality. Both positions are markedly different from my example of Ana, who did not hate her father but who also did not try to excuse or justify what he had done. This was perhaps what helped her ultimately to separate from him psychically.

The most outspoken child of a Nazi perpetrator has been Niklas Frank, who published an excoriating account of his father, *Der Vater*, in 1987. As Hitler's personal lawyer, Hans Frank rose to power and became chief jurist in occupied Poland from 1939 to 1941, where he was known for his reign of terror over the civilian population, establishing Jewish ghettos and responsible for the mass murder of Jews. Niklas describes his father as narcissistic, distant and at times cruel. His parents' relationship was fraught, both greedy for power and wealth. Niklas's memories of his childhood include being driven with his mother in the family's chauffeured car while his mother raided the Jewish shops for discounted luxury goods. His childhood comes across as lonely, harsh and frightening. He describes his father as a "weak" man. Referring to his father's change of plea to guilty during the Nuremberg Trial, Niklas commented, "His true character emerged with that second statement" (Sands, p.362). The fact that his father was accused and ultimately hung following the Nuremberg verdict, for crimes against humanity, seems to underscore Niklas's pre-existing hatred of his father. He did not have to reconcile contradictory realities; he had one father whose behavior was relatively consistent at home and at work. Niklas's repudiation of his father could be complete. As he said about his father in a television interview, "Having your neck broken spared me from having a screwed-up life. How you would have poisoned me with your brainwashing, just like they did to the silent majority of my generation – those not lucky enough to have had their father hanged" (Hitler's Children, 2012).

Another tortured scion of the Nazi legacy is Rainer Hoess, grandson of Rudolf Hoess and nephew to Ingebirgitt. The stigma of his grandfather's crimes has taken on an ontological meaning in his life. He asks, "Why am I alive? To carry this guilt, this burden, to try to come to terms with it? I think that must be the only reason I exist" (Hitler's Children, 2012). And yet when the grandson Hoess describes memories of his own father, we can begin to see some of the foundations for his bitterness. He explains,

> There was no warmth between my father and us. Never. He told us what to do and we obeyed. He set the rules and we obeyed. My father never let us show weakness, show emotion. He hated that to death. Whenever we cried, we were beaten even more, just for crying, not for what we had done … He remained a zealot of the Third Reich.
>
> (Hitler's Children)

Rainer Hoess's burden of guilt seems to be proportionate to his hatred of his father and, ultimately, of his grandfather's deeds.

Others, who did not have such hostile relationships with their fathers, nevertheless chose to go into hiding and to distance themselves from their pasts. Ingebirgitt Hoess never used her father's name, even on her mother's gravestone, for fear of reprisals, explaining, "There are crazy people out there. They might burn my house down or shoot somebody" (Harding, 2013). Ingebirgitt Hoess also finds it hard to believe the full horror of her father's crimes, asking, "How can there be so many survivors if so many had been killed?" (Harding, 2013). Bettina Goering, Hermann Goering's grand-niece, emigrated from Germany to New Mexico to start a new life. Both she and her brother had themselves sterilized to ensure that their family line would be killed off, curiously, and perhaps unconsciously, repeating the Nazi drive for racial sterilization of the Jews as a way of cleansing the Aryan population of contaminating elements. Even though she was born after the war, Bettina Goering claims, "I feel responsible for the Holocaust … because of my family, who had an active part in it" (Hitler's Children).

Gudrun Himmler, daughter of Heinrich Himmler, architect of the Final Solution, also went into hiding, marrying and assuming her husband's name and keeping her family identity secret. Like Ingebirgitt Hoess, Gudrun Himmler may have gone into hiding out of fear of reprisal. She continues to assert her father's innocence of genocide. Her efforts to care for her father's former associates along with her active participation in the NPD (Nationalistiche Partei Deutschlands), the right-wing German Nationalist Party, suggest that she has remained loyal to ideology of the Reich (Lebert & Lebert, 2000, p.13).

While Gudrun Himmler kept her connections to the past alive but secret, other Nazi children demonstrated their loyalty to their fathers by immersing themselves in their fathers' histories in an attempt to defend and vindicate their crimes. Wolf Rüdiger Hess, son of Rudolf Hess, spent most of his life arguing for an investigation of his father's death, claiming the British Secret Service had murdered him in order to prevent his parole and the disclosure of embarrassing information about the British Secret Service. Hess's argument was incontrovertibly refuted in 2007 (six years after Hess's death) by the publication of documents that clearly demonstrated British support for Rudolf Hess's parole. Before his death, Wolf Rüdiger, stressed, "I never had any time. I spent all my free time on my father" (Lebert & Lebert, p.76). Hess's compulsion to defend his father suggests that his own narcissistic identification was at stake. Niklas Frank observes, "There are two ways to survive for a child of a war criminal – to defend him until the end like my older brothers or to confront with his actions and to admit, 'Yes, our father was a criminal'" (Hitler's Children). Confronting the truth is inevitably more difficult because of its narcissistic implications. The Leberts argue that the Nazi children who failed to disavow their fathers also claim to have benefitted from their fathers' legacies. They comment,

> There seems to be a connection there: a child that so passionately deifies its father draws from his pretended significance and one-time lustre a considerable part of its own sense of itself – and is simultaneously incapable of owning up that its family history is, in truth, a serious psychological handicap.
>
> (Lebert & Lebert, p.213)

The Leberts explain the need amongst some Nazi children to deny their tainted family history as a defense against their own narcissistic injury. For many Nazi children, such as Ingebirgitt Hoess, it is important to remember that their childhood was lived in the reflected glory of their fathers, many of whom were highly admired and revered amongst their peers. They were Hitler's blessed children. With the failure of the Reich and, worse still, with the arrests and imprisonment of their fathers, these children experienced a sudden and devastating loss of grace. Ingebirgitt Hoess describes the British search for her father at the end of the war:

> I remember when they came to our house to ask questions. I was sitting on the table with my sister. I was about 13 years old. The British soldiers were screaming: 'Where is your father? Where is your father?' over and over again. I got a very bad headache. I went outside and cried under a tree. I made myself calm down. I made myself stop crying, and my headache went away ...
>
> (Harding, 2013)

As another daughter of an SS officer succinctly put it, "I was a nobody now" (Children of the Third Reich).

Katrin Himmler, Heinrich Himmler's great-niece, like Niklas Frank, has chosen to acknowledge publicly her family connections and history as a way of coming to terms with her past. In her documentary, *Family Members of Heinrich Himmler*, Katrin states,

In our family, it was useful to have this evil personified in Heinrich Himmler, the culmination of all evil. All the others could easily fade into his shadow. This had an impact on the family, and still does for some, so that for a long time no one examined what the other family members had done. Heinrich eased the burden for the rest of us.

(Hitler's Children)

In another interview, Katrin admits to feeling sick when she discovered her grandmother had been a Nazi.

Katrin has perhaps been able to explore her past so openly because, unlike many other Nazi families, the history of her family was spoken about. She recalls,

My father told us about the family constellation very early on, he spoke openly about the fact that Heinrich Himmler was his uncle, his god-father even, and that he had committed terrible crimes. As a young child it was clear to me how difficult this was. How emotionally difficult this was for him and therefore for us, to be related to this mass murderer. I remember it as an emotional burden. When we were children, my sister and I thought it was good that only girls were in our family, so that the name of Himmler would eventually die out. We wanted the name to disappear or be erased.

(Hitler's Children)

Katrin makes it clear that she wanted her name to "disappear" out of shame. In contrast to Bettina Goering, Katrin asserts, "I was never afraid that in my genes there is 'the bad blood from Heinrich Himmler.' I think that if I believed that, then I would be upholding the Nazi theories that everything is genetically determined" (Hitler's Children).[6] In acknowledging what for so many German families could not be spoken about, Katrin seems to have accepted her history and the crimes committed by her family and society, without being crippled by it.

My patient, Ana, began to accept her own tie to her father's crimes when she became aware of her disfigured left hand in her dream. Seeing this grotesque part of herself allowed her to realize that, while she was like her father, she could be different from him. Katrin comments, "There came a point when I felt I could live with this name. But I wanted my son to have the chance to start again, to have this different name. That's different than giving up a name that is part of your life" (Family members of Heinrich Himmler).

Transgenerational Guilt

For the children of perpetrators who deny their father's crimes, there is no consequent guilt to contend with.[7] Just as the crime is disavowed so is the guilt attached to it. This is not the case for those children who acknowledge their fathers' crimes, like Niklas Frank, Rainer Hoess and Katrin Himmler, who are faced with the burden of guilt by association. As Niklas Frank asserts, "Yes, I feel responsible for my father's actions and I'm ashamed for this."

Shame and guilt are interwoven. There is the contamination attached to the proximity of evil that imbues shame. Primo Levi describes this in the faces of the Russian soldiers as they liberated Auschwitz and witnessed the atrocities that had taken place:

> They did not greet us, nor smile; they seemed oppressed, not only by pity but also by a confused restraint which sealed their mouths, and kept their eyes fastened on the funereal scene. It was the same shame which we knew so well, which submerged us after the selections, and every time we had to witness or undergo an outrage: the shame that the Germans never knew, the shame which the just man experiences when confronted by a crime committed by another, and he feels remorse because of its existence, because of its having been irrevocably introduced into the world of existing things, and because his will has proven non-existent or feeble and was incapable of putting up a good defence.
>
> (Levi, 1989, p.54)

Levi starkly points out that it was the victims and the observers who experienced shame, not the Germans. This highlights the fact that there was no place in the system of the camps, or indeed within the administration responsible for devising and implementing the Final Solution, for shame or guilt as this would signify a deep flaw at the heart of the Reich's ideology. The totalist belief system ascribed to by most Nazi officers was consistent within its own particular closed world. This, more than anything else, explains why so many of the Nazi war criminals did not plead guilty when brought to trial. Although Hans Frank changed his plea at the end of his trial, Niklas scoffed at his father's confession of guilt, assuming this was a kind of safeguard or deal his father was making with God to save face. However, this initial failure to acknowledge guilt on the part of those who had committed the crimes was the principal cause of the damage suffered by the next generation in Germany. Unacknowledged guilt was passed on to the children, left to atone for the deeds passed on to them from their fathers and to untangle the remnants of a perverse belief system that had corrupted everyone's lives.[8]

The guilt experienced by the children of perpetrators is not only the consequence of being left to deal with the sins of their fathers, for those children who loved their parents were also left with another form of guilt – that of loving someone who is tainted by evil. In his novel, *The Reader*, Schlink writes about a young German boy's coming of age love affair with an older woman, Hanna, who suddenly, and inexplicably, disappears at a time when he was beginning to have his own, separate life from her. It is only years later, as a student attending a war trial, that the narrator discovers to his horror that the woman he loved is there in front of him, standing trial for her acts as an SS officer in a concentration camp. It becomes clear in the course of Hanna's trial that she fails to defend herself because, he realizes, defending herself would mean revealing her illiteracy. It was more important to her to keep this a secret than to deny charges that she had issued written orders for the killings of prisoners. The narrator understands,

> She accepted that she would be called to account, and simply did not wish to endure further exposure. She was not pursuing her own interests, but fighting for her own truth, her own justice.
>
> (Schlink, 1997, pp.132–3)

The narrator then has to confront his guilt for a series of betrayals; his betrayal in pushing Hanna away when he was young and beginning to be interested in other things in his life, his betrayal in deciding not to reveal to the court that she was illiterate, a fact that would have spared her a life sentence, and, finally, his guilt in "having loved a criminal" (Schlink, 1997, p.133).[6] The poignancy of the story lies in the symbol of illiteracy. Although at the time of the Third Reich Germany had the highest literacy rate in Europe, illiteracy signifies the ignorance that allowed ordinary people to become swept up in committing atrocities. Another interpretation of Hanna's illiteracy is that it represents the Third Reich's "moral illiteracy" (Wroe, 2002), something even more shaming, and hence to be kept hidden, than the acts to which this gave rise.

Hoffman addresses the dilemma expressed by Schlink of "loving a criminal" and the predicament of being in what she refers to as a "no-win position". Hoffman writes,

> ... for to remain fixed in hatred and fear of one's parents, one's first objects of love, is to risk emotional stultification, or even death. But to give in to impulses of attachment and affection, when they are directed towards parents who have committed horrific crimes, and who have done so not out of passion but from conviction and belief – to accept this is surely to give up a part of one's own moral being.
>
> (Hoffman, p.122)

However, what Schlink's narrator shows us is quite the reverse. He has not given up his own moral being in continuing to love this woman, he has in fact confirmed his moral being through his own awareness of his betrayals and his guilt. Hoffman seems to be confusing accepting the reality of evil with condoning it while the two are very different. Not to accept is to perpetuate a psychological splitting and denial that gives credence to the idea that evil can be located outside us, if not eradicated altogether.

Restorative Guilt and False Guilt

Children of perpetrators carry not only their own family histories but also the history of their communities. By virtue of their close association to evil, children of perpetrators are at the forefront in being forced to find a way of living with extreme moral contradictions that many of us do not have to confront in our everyday lives. In their study of the children of Nazi leaders, the Leberts question whether they have "become a kind of lightning conductor for German history?" (Lebert & Lebert, p.76). Certainly they have played an important role as receptacles and scapegoats for collective guilt. However, this is also a role that, at least potentially, carries social influence and transformation. For many children, acknowledging the crimes of their fathers, especially in light of the denial expressed by so many perpetrators, can also be understood as a means of restoring a sense of moral order. The commission of an atrocity, or an act that intends to dehumanize a person, forces us to recognize that something outside the bounds of our perceived social norms has occurred. Our immediate sense of social and moral order is turned upside-down and fundamentally threatened. The world that we can count on and, in most instances, trust no longer exists. This creates a state of anomie, taken from the Greek "anomia" meaning lawlessness. On a social and collective level, the acknowledgement of wrongdoing affirms that harm has been done, that someone is responsible, that there is concern for the injured person, and that something destructive has happened that may not necessarily be possible to repair but needs to be acknowledged and mourned, at least on a personal level. Through this acknowledgement, the tenets of both a social and moral order are restored and re-confirmed. The shame experienced by children of perpetrators both enables and is the process by which they can restore a sense of moral order and integrity within their families and for the future. This is similarly so on a collective level.

Our acknowledgement of wrongdoing and collective responsibility not only protects us from the threat of anomie, it also serves as a reminder of the past and keeps our ability to observe and judge alive. The act of remembering in itself performs a cathartic function as it validates our experienced reality and enables us to separate past from present. Imre Kertész, in writing about the Holocaust, stresses the necessity to remember and to have a history in order to go on being a person. However painful the memory is, it brings with it the knowledge that we are responsible towards ourselves and others. Kertész exclaims,

> 'No!' something bellows, howls, within me, I don't wish to remember, ... remembering is knowing, we live in order to remember what we know, because we cannot forget what we know, ... we are not able, to forget, that is the way we are created ... the reason why we know and remember

is in order that somebody should feel shame on our account ... *in any case you're always partly to blame.*

(Kertész, 2004, pp.26–7)

Kertész conversely warns us that without memory, there is no one to blame. This is the plight of children who deny the crimes their fathers have committed and, in doing so, deny a part of themselves, their own self-agency. In this respect, guilt helps to protect us from dissociating from our past and from ourselves. Guilt preserves our humanity.

While it is evident that guilt serves a variety of important functions, it can also be used in a malignant or false way, becoming a kind of politically correct smokescreen that actually hides other ills. The young narrator in Schlink's novel describes his peers' blanket condemnation of their parents simply because they had been of the generation of the Third Reich. Despite the fact that his father had lost his job as a philosophy professor on political grounds, the son condemned both his parents "to shame". The narrator admits, "We all condemned our parents to shame, even if the only charge we could bring was that after 1945 they had tolerated the perpetrators in their midst" (Schlink, 1997, p.90). But the narrator's shame, or guilt, in this regard is conveyed as a reaction conforming to the zeitgeist of his time. He notes the feigned interest expressed by his fellow students in the horrors of the Holocaust,

When I think about it now, I think that our eagerness to assimilate the horrors and our desire to make everyone else aware of them was in fact repulsive. The more horrible the events about which we read and heard, the more certain we became of our responsibility to enlighten and accuse. Even when the facts took our breath away, we held them up triumphantly. Look at this!

(Schlink, 1997, p.91)

The students are filled with the self-righteousness of the converted; their eagerness to acknowledge guilt belies their disavowal of it.

During the trial of his lover, Schlink's narrator comments on the "general numbness" that seemed to take hold of perpetrators, victims, judges, members of the court and others attending. "When I likened perpetrators, victims, the dead, the living, survivors, and their descendants to each other, I didn't feel good about it and I still don't" (Schlink, 1997, p.101). Kertész's phrase, we are all "partly to blame", does not mean that we can all be likened to one another and in this way erase the horror and the significance of the distinctions between us.

A number of the children of perpetrators have been recorded as saying that they wish their own lives could be taken in expiation of the deaths caused by their fathers. They are expressing not only a wish to absolve themselves of their own associated guilt but also a primitive notion of social justice – an eye for an eye – in the hope that one death would cancel out the other. But underlying the idea that they deserve such retribution, is the wish to be recognized as a victim too. The difference between perpetrator and victim can then be ignored and the child of the perpetrator can become an honorable victim rather than a person dirtied by his father's past. It is a form of narcissistic masochism that washes clean the sadism that is perceived as dangerous and taboo.

Hoffman distinguishes this kind of extreme guilt as a form of "pseudo-identification with Jewish victims". In describing a patient, the daughter of SS parents, Hoffman writes,

> She felt she was like them; she wanted to know Jews and feel close to them. This, too, is a theme that surfaces in German second-generation literature, and it is a delicate and troubling one. Sympathy for the victim and a reparative urge are the decent responses in genocide's wake. But the desire to impersonate or appropriate the identity of the other in order to disburden oneself of one's own carries with it the risk of inauthenticity and the seeds of bad faith ... in stories like this ... we can find clues as to the roots of that wider identification with the victim that has been such a prominent feature of postwar German politics.
>
> (Hoffman, p.123)

These are examples of how guilt can be misread and perverted into bad faith, motivated by and disguising narcissistic needs. Like the students in Schlink's novel, it is the triumph of the self-righteous that negates genuine guilt.

The Irresolvable Conflict of Evil

A son of a Nazi perpetrator reads his father's last words to his mother before being hanged,

> "I swear I never ordered or committed a crime." The son remarks in disgust, "... how many lies? ... Of course he's lying, or he can't see what he did as a crime ... because he sees himself as just a tool – that's particularly awful for me. I've read his statement of defense. In it, he describes the Gestapo as a normal administrative body with normal tasks. That was even more shocking for me because it was such a stupid argument. He seems to have had such a naïve attitude to this system. I was really shocked. I would almost have preferred a cleverer father. It's shaming ..."
>
> (Children of the Third Reich)

And how unbearable to have had a father who was so blind to what was going on and his part in it. But the son also assumes that if his father had been "cleverer", he would have been different. Unfortunately, this is far from the case. The problem of the Reich was that what wasn't "normal" could not simply be attributed to the stupidity, sadism or madness of its administrators – there is plenty of evidence to show that the SS cannot simply be classified as monsters and madmen. And the son's reaction to his father's professed innocence goes deeper than shame and loss of respect, there is also his disbelief that points to something that is unthinkable about what his father did. And by virtue of the fact that it was his *father*, what does this mean about him?

The legacy that these children, along with my patient, Ana, have inherited is precisely this struggle to make sense of how such evil could have happened without attributing it to a single cause and therefore something we can process mentally that is in some way familiar. The experience of evil is that it is *unthinkable*, it is not only beyond the bounds of our everyday existence, it is antithetical to the world we know, it is a world that is *ahuman*.[9] Because evil destroys our social norms it is by its very nature hard to integrate in our thinking and in our experience of life. This is true for all of us, but especially so for people who have been touched by evil – victims and the families of perpetrators. Trust in a seemingly predictable and consistent reality is shattered and, even more importantly, trust in those we are closest to and most dependent on is thrown into doubt. Niklas Frank, speaking to a German audience, warns,

> I don't trust any of you. Who knows? If the economy turns bad again, you might get those ideas again, to follow a strong leader, restrict ethnic minorities, maybe even imprison them. You don't have to call it "concentration camps". Here and there you have a little murder, a little killing. It might help purify the bloodline. Besides, it will create more jobs for the real Germans.
>
> (Hitler's Children)

How close our realpolitik is coming to this now.

What is most disturbing for children of perpetrators and what they are acutely aware of because of their close links to evil, is that the kernel of evil does not reside in others, it resides in all of us. We are all born with the mark of Cain. Niklas Frank conveys the anguish of his identification with his father when he says, "I'm sure I've hated (him) so very much because I kept finding him in myself" (Lebert & Lebert, p.16). Ana's dream image of her atrophied left hand also signified her identification with a father who had kept hidden a lifeless and life-destroying part of himself. Both Niklas and Ana could only hate this aspect of themselves and yet it was their hatred that allowed them to acknowledge and incorporate the presence of evil within themselves.

The experience and proximity of evil is contaminating and disorienting; it is also alienating. The children of perpetrators share with victims the knowledge of a ruptured world, a loss of innocence that can never be regained. There is an initial shock that numbs the capacity for memory or piecing together the two strange realities of past and present. Patrick Modiano describes this state of mind in postwar France,

> I told myself that nobody remembers anything anymore ... And yet from time to time, beneath this thick layer of amnesia, you can certainly sense something, an echo, distant, muted, but of what, precisely, it is impossible to say. Like finding yourself on the edge of a magnetic field, with no pendulum to pick up the radiation.
>
> (Modiano, 2014, pp.124–5)

Those who try to resolve the contradictions left in the wake of evil by expelling or masking the truth continue to live in a twilight world without a center. Paradoxically, it is the act of remembering and what this entails that centers us and allows us to create a different future.

Notes

1 An abridged version of this paper first appeared in the British Journal of Psychotherapy, February 2018, vol. 34 no. 1.
2 See Fromm, M.G., ed., (2012). *Lost in Transmission: Studies of Trauma Across Generations*. London: Karnac. Fonagy, P. "The transgenerational transmission of Holocaust trauma." Chap 20 in. Eds. Covington, C., Williams, P., Arundale, J. and Knox, J. *Terrorism and War: Unconscious Dynamics of Political Violence*. London: Karnac. Volkan, V. (2006). *Killing in the Name of Identity*. Charlottesville, Virginia: Pitchstone Publishing.
3 See Sichrovsky, P. (1988). *Born Guilty: Children of Nazi Families*. New York: Basic Books. Bar-On, D. (1989). *Legacy of Silence: Encounters with Children of the Third Reich*. Cambridge, Massachusetts: Harvard University Press. See also *Children of the Third Reich*, a film produced by Catrine Clay, BBC2, 10th November 1993.
4 Studies of families of violent offenders demonstrate that they often experience associative shame, ostracism, and victimization. See Condry, R. (2007). *Families Shamed: The Consequences of Crime for Relatives of Serious Offenders*. London: Routledge.
5 Nazi perpetrators were most commonly men, but women were also actively involved in committing atrocities, either as Nazi officers or as adjutants to their Nazi husbands. See Lower, W. (2013). *Hitler's Furies: German Women in the Nazi Killing Fields*. London: Chatto & Windus.
6 The thrust of Hitler's vision of the Reich and the new German supremacy was to recreate the purity of the Aryan race.
7 I do not mean to suggest here that children of perpetrators are guilty of their parents' crimes but that they must find a way not only of living with their feelings about their parents but also dealing with the social stigma and accusations of guilt by proxy.
8 In commenting on the conflicting belief systems evident in post-war Germany, Hoffman writes: "the public climate in which the younger German grew up was diametrically opposed to the belief system of their parents. Indeed, Peter Sichrovksy interestingly suggests that the contradictions between what he calls a 'fascistic

family structure' and the post-war democratic ethos both increased the tensions between the generations and ultimately enabled the young to rebel against the parents and break the bonds that tied them to the past." (Hoffman, p.124)

9 For an account on the nature of evil and its effects on us see Covington, C. (2016). "Do we need a theory of evil?" In *Everyday Evils: A Psychoanalytic View of Evil and Morality*. London: Routledge.

References

Bachmann, I. (2018). *War Diary*. London: Seagull.

Bar-On, D. (1999). *The Indescribable and the Undiscussable: Reconstructing Human Discourse after Trauma*. Budapest: Central European University Press.

"*Children of the Third Reich*". Produced by Catrine Clay for BBC2, first shown on 10 November 1993.

Hall, A. (1 June 2015). "'My beautiful Auschwitz childhood': Daughter of camp commandant Rudolph Hoess describes life growing up next to a concentration camp – and how she has hidden her identity for decades." *MailOnline*.

Harding, T. (7 September 2013). "Hiding in N. Virginia, a daughter of Auschwitz." *Washington Post*.

Himmler, K. (19 June 2012). "*Family members of Heinrich Himmler*". Documentary film available on www.docsonline.tv.

"*Hitler's Children*". Produced by Chanoch Zeevi, first shown on Israeli Channel 2 on 1st May 2011, and on BBC2 in 2012.

Hoffman, E. (2004). *After Such Knowledge*. London: Vintage.

Kertesz, I. (2004) *Kaddish for an Unborn Child*. London: Random House.

Lebert, S. & Lebert, N. (2000). *My Father's Keeper: Children of Nazi Leaders – An Intimate History of Damage and Denial*. London: Little, Brown and Company.

Levi, P. (1989). *The Drowned and the Saved*. London: Abacus.

McGlothlin, E. (2006). *Second-Generation Holocaust Literature: Legacies of Survival and Perpetration*. London: Camden House.

Modiano, P. (2014). *The Search Warrant*. London: Harvill Secker.

Sands, P. (2016). *East West Street*. London: Weidenfeld & Nicolson.

Schlink, B. (1997). *The Reader*. London: Phoenix.

Schlink, B. (2012). "Johann Sebastian Bach on Ruegen." In *Summer Lies*. London: Phoenix.

Sicher, E. ed. (1998). *Breaking Crystal: Writing and Memory after Auschwitz*. Urbana, Illinois: University of Illinois Press.

Wroe, N. (9 February 2002). "Reader's guide to a moral maze." *The Guardian*.

Chapter 3

Collective Guilt – a Moral Imperative?

> When we all know what's going on, each of us can hide in the shadows.
>
> (Patrick, banker)

Introduction

In Judeo-Christian culture, the confession and atonement for committing sins brings us back to God and restores social purity. Prior to the Holocaust, there are many historical examples across the world of atrocities committed on racial groups under the power of foreign empires or in the commercial enterprise of slavery. The Holocaust marked a turning point in the world's moral consciousness, bringing about the use of the word "genocide" and its meaning. For the first time in history, war crimes were viewed in a different light. The Nuremberg Trials held after the end of World War Two initiated legal recognition of individuals responsible for war crimes and crimes against humanity. Subsequent trials in Germany and the institution of the International Criminal Court of Justice at The Hague continue to hold individuals accountable for war crimes. These tribunals, however, do not determine the collective guilt of a nation. They can only determine individual guilt. And yet, throughout history, the finger of guilt is pointed at nations and groups that have been responsible for the persecution and deaths of others, especially at the point when these groups have been defeated.

If we look at postwar Germany as an example, the liberation of the concentration camps by the Allies was almost immediately followed by Allied programs aimed at inducing guilt and shame in the German population.[1] Queues of German citizenry were filmed as they were forced by the Allies to enter the camps and to witness the sites of mass killing. Not surprisingly, we also see many of the Germans denying that they ever knew such things had gone on and so near to where they lived. There is increasing evidence that many Germans, particularly those living in proximity to concentration camps, did know about the persecution and cruelties inflicted on the Jews and other targeted minorities.[2] But when faced with heaps of emaciated corpses in the

DOI: 10.4324/9781003379980-4

camps under Allied surveillance, were these German witnesses really going to confess they had known all along? Looking back, and without condoning the practices of the Reich, this looks like a mass exercise in humiliation and shame. These programs were a clear expression of the moral imperative imposed on the German population from the Allies that they should take on the mantle of guilt as a nation for the evils that had been committed under the Reich.

While the Allies did not question the "rightness" of pointing the finger of collective guilt at the Germans, and indeed many Germans today agree on the importance of atoning for their guilt, the historical evidence of the German population *experiencing* actual guilt is complex and arguable. This also applies to other countries, such as Poland, Rwanda and Serbia, in which public displays of mourning over genocidal killings take on different meanings depending on the political and historical context.

In this chapter I will focus on the experience and history of Germany at the end of the Third Reich and subsequently. Not only is there now a wealth of historical material but, within this, detailed personal accounts that give us new insights into the complexities of guilt and shame that were experienced by some, but by no means all, Germans. Causes of guilt and shame also varied and were not all related to the atrocities committed under the regime. The shame of defeat was particularly evident along with the hardships of postwar life. While in my previous chapter I wrote about the experience of many children of high-ranking Nazi officers and their personal struggle to come to terms with the crimes of their parents, their experience does not necessarily reflect or imply a collective experience of guilt.

Guilty for What?

Postwar Germany, with the division of East and West, is a particularly striking example of the extent to which collective guilt featured after partition and the role it played in forming the identity and political future of each zone. Guilt does not exist in a vacuum but within a social context in which certain acts are considered crimes. In the case of Germany, we find markedly different reactions and interpretations of guilt that arose in West Germany and East Germany. It is questionable that immediately following the end of the war, whether in West or East Germany, guilt was a predominant or even noticeable feature of the social psyche. Those of us from Allied nations forget the trauma suffered by the Germans at the end of the war and in the hardship of recovery.

German soldiers returning from the war were under no illusion of what defeat would mean, particularly cognizant of fear of reprisals from the Russians and punitive measures from the Allies. The German narrator in a fictional account of the war recounts:

> There was a joke that was now always trotted out whenever someone complained: "Enjoy the war, the peace will be much worse." It always

made me think of my school Latin, and the story about Rome being sacked by Brennus the Gaul. The Romans had agreed to pay Brennus to leave the city. When they were weighing out the stipulated price in gold and silver, they complained that the scales were rigged against them. Brennus threw his sword on top, making it worse, and said, *Vae victis*, woe to the conquered. That's what it means to be at someone's mercy.

(Starritt, 2020, Loc. 554–9)

Many Germans whose families and lives had been destroyed by the war felt embittered and saw themselves as the victimized group – especially those who had believed in the vision of the Reich. One young woman describes clearing up the damage in Berlin immediately following the end of the war:

Carry debris to the mountain of rubble in the W Strasse at six in the morning. Row of buckets. We had to work very hard. I was there with Lotte Martin. She was there because her father had been a party member. I was home at 10pm. That's sixteen hours of hard work. If it goes on like this many of the women won't be able to continue. It's dreadful, how us Germans have to demean ourselves.

(Berlin 1945, Brigitte Eicke, Episode 3)[3]

An American correspondent voiced the Allied condemnation of the Germans: "I'm afraid the Germans have still not learnt the lesson of this terrible war. They're only sorry for themselves – not for all those they murdered and tortured and tried to wipe from the face of the earth." (Berlin 1945, William L. Shirer, Episode 3) From a different perspective, a Red Army lieutenant admitted: "Many of my acquaintances, friends even, will think that I am touched, that I fell for the German citizen, the German population. I have to confess, no. I will never ever pity them since I have seen for myself the havoc they have caused in Russia" (Berlin 1945, Konrad Wolf, Episode 2).

The stigmatization of the Germans as a group not only ignored the silent dissenters and those who were trapped within a belief system they could not alter, but it also conveniently ignored the fact that the Allies themselves had been slow to intervene while being cognizant of these same atrocities. Foreign observers were anxious to distance themselves from the atrocities they witnessed, as if having any kind of understanding, much less sympathy, of how the Germans had come to this would contaminate them. As a result, few foreigners could fathom the humiliation many Germans felt at the end of the war as their own survival was at stake. A German group analyst, Regine Scholz, comments,

In West Germany no one wanted to face the past. What was most important was to build the future and to make repairs after the war – guilt was not in the social conscience or discourse. It was perhaps not so much a question of denial, but more of dissociation; people did not want to be reminded of the past – of their crimes, their failures, their narcissistic pleasures nor of their losses, hardships and traumas. Many did not have the psychic capacity to confront this complex past, instead "deciding" not to feel anything, thus being in a state of numbness that only allowed people to focus on everyday life in the present.

(Personal communication)

There were also others who thought they had done what was right at the time and found it hard to grasp how it could have ended so disastrously.

Collective guilt became a survival tool in West Germany's attempts to get back on its feet economically. Ironically, the huge push in industrialization fostered the assimilation of business and political leaders who had been active Nazi officials or sympathizers. In building trade and political relations with the West, West Germans demonstrated their collective guilt in memorials and museums as an attempt to cleanse themselves before foreign eyes. De-nazification was promoted through assimilation and atonement. Acceptance of social guilt was the entry ticket to a liberal, democratic society.[4] The public displays of remorse and responsibility for the Nazi past by West Germany further strengthened its alliance with the West against communism. In contrast, East Germany, as a communist, anti-fascist state, wanted to purge itself of Nazi members; e.g., trials against former Nazis were much more numerous and sentences much harsher than in the West.[5] However, for East Germany this had more to do with upholding a new communist system in which the fascist Nazis had committed crimes against the state rather than coming from a need to be absolved of guilt for atrocities. Many communists had been persecuted under Hitler, including Erich Honecker who had been a political prisoner for ten years, and the establishment of the German Democratic Republic enabled them to return to power. In this respect, the losses incurred by the war were mitigated, if not transformed into victory, in East Germany by the empowerment of communism and anti-fascist ideology. Amongst West Germans, loss was defended against by means of strengthening industrialization and ties with the West.

The historian, Mary Fulbrook, writes about the different cultures in East and West Germany that led to very different perceptions of the past.

More generally, younger generations in the GDR could readily understand and empathize with parents or grandparents who had been members of the Nazi party ... young people ... had little choice about joining the state youth groups, mass organizations, the ruling SED, or one of the allied bloc parties. In the light of their own experiences of conformity and coercion, with significant penalties for trying to stand out against what was expected of them, they sympathized with grandparents or parents who said this had also been the case in the Third Reich. Their school education as well as the "antifascist myth" also relieved them of any burden of inherited guilt.

(Fulbrook, 2018, p.452)

East Germans born after the war were far less likely than West Germans of the same generation either to have a sense of connection with the Nazi past or to argue that it was time to "put a line under it"; they were simply less concerned with it in any way at all. Many of the issues of the "second generation" in perpetrator families were specific to West Germans socialized in an atmosphere where a sense of national responsibility for a shameful past was prevalent, indeed inescapable. For East Germans, the turning point of 1989–90, with the collapse of communist rule and the disappearance of the GDR, was a far more significant event than the war.

(Fulbrook, p.453)

Certain achievements made under the GDR, such as improvements for women in employment and more progressive laws for abortion, were not recognized in the West. East Germans could not get equivalent jobs or did not feel valued for what they had done with the result that there was a great sense of loss, envy and hatred towards the West. Reunification was experienced amongst East Germans as a profound disappointment, making them feel like second-class citizens and shattering dreams of a better life.

Historically, there were other significant differences between East and West Germany that influenced their respective experiences. East Germany relied on a feudal economy and social structure with large landowners supporting a poor population of serfs, whereas West Germany had been far more industrialized. This difference meant that the East Germans were much more accustomed to an authoritarian style of government; the feudal system was naturally adaptable to the Nazi system and this in turn to the communist system. The East was motivated to embrace the Nazi regime because it freed them from the elites and their feudal position while at the same time retaining an authoritarian structure. At the end of the war, communist ideology offered the familiarity and continuity of yet another authoritarian structure.

The example of differences between East and West Germany illustrates the complexity of understanding the nature and function of guilt – whether in the individual child of a perpetrator or throughout a generation. Fulbrook highlights the role of socialization and the way in which the past is interpreted as key factors in the framing of guilt on a large scale within a social group. Political and economic differences also make a significant mark on prevailing existential concerns. Guilt arises from a breach of social norms and values, internalized by the group. When the external system of values differs from an internalized system of values, the result is cognitive dissonance, and adaptation to the external system of values is necessary for the survival of the group. This was apparent in West Germany where the external system of values suddenly changed in direct opposition to the previous system of values. In East Germany, the transition from fascism to communism did not create such a stark disjunction; fascism was the predominant crime that needed to be addressed and combatted in the effort to build a strong communist state. As such, the trials of war criminals in East Germany resulted in far stricter punitive measures as they symbolized the communist effort to purge the state of fascist leaders and to protect the state against subversive citizens.[6] In West Germany, war criminals tended to get off more lightly, especially as many were valuable for their experience in industry and useful to the new economy (Fulbrook). John O. Koehler, the German historian, notes:

> Despite widespread misgivings about the judicial failures in connection with Nazi crimes, a number of judges and prosecutors were convicted and jailed for up to three years for perversion of justice. In collusion with the Stasi, they had requested or handed down more severe sentences in political cases so that the state could collect greater amounts when the "convicts" were ransomed by the West German government. (The amount of ransom paid was governed by the time a prisoner had been sentenced to serve.)
>
> (Koehler, 1999)

Along with what defines a crime, the other aspect in determining guilt is that there is a witness to confirm a crime has been committed. The Frankfurt Auschwitz trials of the sixties that took place in West Germany were witnessed by a new generation who were starting to ask their parents what had happened under the Reich. This generation was also exposed to the West and western perceptions of the Reich through travel, which perhaps contributed to a belief that guilt should be expressed on a personal level. East Germans remained relatively isolated and were not so susceptible to social pressure to acknowledge and experience guilt.

The role of the witness – whether it was in western democracies or communism under Soviet rule – determined the nature of the crime itself. The triangulation of perpetrator/victim/witness was enacted in the West specifically by focusing on the crime of genocide.[7] The crime was in the nature of harm done to human rights, both on a collective level and against individuals belonging to the collective. German Foreign Minister Klaus Kinkel, speaking at a session of parliament in September 1991, stressed, "We must punish the perpetrators. This is not a matter of a victor's justice. We owe it to the ideal of justice and to the victims. All of those who ordered injustices and those who executed the orders must be punished; the top men of the SED as well as the ones who shot (people) at the wall." Kinkel continued,

> ... we cannot tolerate that the problems are swept under the rug as a way of dealing with a horrible past, because the results will later be disastrous

for society. We Germans know from our own experience where this leads. Jewish philosophy formulates it in this way: "The secret of redemption is called remembering."

(Koehler, p.14)

Within East Germany, the threat to the future was not located internally, it was externalized and projected onto the "monopoly capitalism" of West Germany, with its links to Nazism. It was not the human rights of the individual that needed to be safeguarded so much as the communist ideology; the individual's interest was aligned if not placed within the totality of the state, as opposed to existing in its own right.

Indoctrination and Betrayal

Without some insight into German culture during the Weimar Republic and the process of indoctrination that occurred at the beginning and throughout the Reich, it is easy to fall into the trap of moralizing or imputing what the Germans felt – or should have felt – when they were defeated. While the victor commonly cites the wrongdoings of the loser as the cause of war, implying that losses suffered are at least in part justified, the expectation that Germans should experience guilt for what had happened under the Reich was particularly pronounced, stigmatizing the German character as evil rather than attempting to understand how the Reich had been able to gain such power.

In a detailed study of German experiences before and after the Reich, Konrad Jarausch, describes the Weimar culture of humiliation in which German children grew up:

> In geography class, the wall maps still contained "the lost territories" and former colonies of the Reich after the "shameful peace of Versailles," instilling resentment ... Even if moderate Social Democrats pleaded for peaceful understanding, many children developed a "sense of offended innocence" in their patriotic commitment ...In many institutions, the legacy of the lost war transformed love of country into a dangerous nationalism, warping young minds. Because they provided all too few ethical grounds for a cosmopolitan humanism, the schools left most of their pupils at the mercy of National Socialist appeals.
>
> (Jarausch, 2018, pp.56–7)

Against this background,

> Helmut Raschdorff remembered that "in 1933 we experienced the so-called seizure of power, which was to bring untold changes that were only feared by a few. In our daily routine at school hardly anything changed" ... Only

gradually did most youths begin to realize that "a terrible time (had begun) when the Nazis gained power."

(Ibid., p.65)

One adolescent girl describes her pleasurable memories of Nazi youth activities and their idealistic appeal. Eva Peters, a youth leader, wrote, "I, too was meant, spoken to and called up to put my life into the service of a great and overpowering (ideal) called Germany." Only later, as she became increasingly aware of the deadly consequences of these nationalistic ideals, was she forced "to seek an explanation of what actually caused for (me) and many other youths of … (my) generation that 'great deception'" (Ibid., p.67). Another young woman wrote, "Searching for comfort, I let myself be captured by a great lie" (Ibid., p.189). These personal accounts convey the seduction and subsequent ambivalence experienced by those who fell prey to the Nazi dream. As a result, Jarausch describes the memory texts as "paradoxical and unstable, drifting from evocative description of enjoyable activities to retrospective condemnation of their catastrophic effect" (Ibid., p.67).

For others, trying to explain their own response to Nazi idealism was more problematic but nevertheless echo the sentiment either that they were being wrongfully blamed or that "we didn't know what we were getting into." Jarausch notes:

> Some apologists such as Karl Hartel resented "the accusations of especially younger people" born after WW II that "it was their generation that was responsible for Hitler having been able to precipitate half of the world into misfortune." Instead, they blamed the victors of WW I for the lack of peace that enabled political dilettantes such as the Nazis to seize power. More self-critical spirits such as Heinz Schultheis cited insufficient age as a reason for their complicity: "For us children these circumstances were an unchangeable condition whose importance we completely failed to recognize; and especially because of that our generation automatically grew into the damned "Third Reich".

(Ibid., p.65)

At the end of the war, those who continued to believe in the Nazi vision felt betrayed by those who condemned the Reich; those who excused or disclaimed their involvement and belief in the regime. On the other hand, the "apologists" and those who had become disillusioned, felt betrayed by the lies they had been told; lies that had not only deprived them of "a normal youth" but had made them culpable of the consequences. One young man

> recalled that patriotic youths slowly realized that they were "willingly or reluctantly participating in a criminal war of incredible dimensions." Hermann Debus remembered how "it gradually dawned upon me, that

'our Fuhrer' had abused us. At any rate, we were no longer convinced of his 'infallibility'. While some fanatics continued to cling to their nationalist faith, many soldiers began to disassociate themselves from the 'damned hoax' of a bankrupt regime."

(Ibid., p.145)[8]

Witnessing and taking part in the monstrous crimes committed in the course of the war became even more unthinkable under "a bankrupt regime". Perpetrators and victims alike not only wanted to repress their experience but to dissociate themselves from it as much as possible.[9]

In addition to feeling betrayed by their leaders, many young people came to feel betrayed by their parents and adult role models who had encouraged their children to follow their idealistic beliefs (Jarausch, p. 95). The ultimate betrayal, however, came with Hitler's suicide on 30th April 1945. One young woman admits that she was "utterly bewildered and confused" when Hitler killed himself. Her response was to join a suicide pact with other young people; she decided she wanted to live and never succeeded (Jarausch, p.179). The idea of suicide was motivated by a variety of factors. In the case of this young woman, it may well have been a powerful expression of loyalty to the ideals that had been smashed at the end of the war, a kind of heroic sacrifice that maintained the belief in Hitler's purity.

However, the shocking exposure of atrocities committed both within Germany and against its enemies abroad was increasingly difficult to deny and inflicted a deeper sense of betrayal that led to mistrust of any belief system and of the dangers of blind faith. Renate Finckh described this as "a terrible recognition: Whatever I had loyally tried to keep in my heart had changed into remorse and shame" (Ibid., p.186). One journalist and loyal Nazi confessed, "I can't carry on ... Everything I believed in is turning out to be madness and crime" (Huber, 2019, p.77).

Mass Suicide

The end of the Reich was marked by three distinct waves of mass suicide. In early January 1945, following the defeat of the Germans by Soviet forces in East Prussia and Silesia, many Germans resorted to suicide out of fear of reprisals and anxiety about their future. Three months later, the Battle of Berlin marked the final defeat of the Third Reich and the end of the Nazi vision. Military personnel, government officials and civilians began committing suicide *en masse*. Hitler and his supporters had encouraged Germans everywhere to fight to the end rather than accept defeat;[10] Hitler's suicide therefore marked that the end had come and, with it, the loss of hope. High-ranking Nazi officials, notably, Joseph Goebbels, Heinrich Himmler, Philipp Bouhler and Martin Bormann, followed suit. In Berlin alone, in April 1945, 3,881 Germans killed themselves.[11] Further waves of suicide across the whole of Germany occurred in the weeks after the end of the war and the takeover by the Allies. Demmin, a small town in Western Pomerania, is particularly well known as the site of between 700 to 1000 suicides in just over three days at the end of April 1945. The suicides in Demmin represented a cross-section of the local population in terms of age, class and profession and as such has been portrayed as a microcosm of suicides being committed across the country.

Different theories have been applied to explain this phenomenon. As German psychiatrist, Erich Menninger-Lerchenthal, observed, "organised mass suicide on a large scale ... had previously not occurred in the history of Europe ... there are suicides which do not have anything to do with mental illness or some moral and intellectual deviance, but predominantly with the continuity of a heavy political defeat and the fear of being held responsible" (Goeschel, 2009, p.165). The Catholic writer, Reinhold Schneider, argued that the suicides signified a culture that had lost its bearings and had strayed from traditional religious values, explaining that "suicide is the certain symbol of the confusion of all order, and it means sin and outrage" (Ibid.). Schneider views suicide as the result of a perverse social order established under the Reich, as a kind of Faustian pact made by the German people to obtain power and supremacy at all costs. There was no way to carry on living once this pact had ended so disastrously. There was also no future left as the Reich could not survive the death of its leader – Hitler's promise of a holy suicide indicates that he himself had no vision of a future in which he was not in charge. The breakdown of the Nazi belief system and the vacuum it left created a certain degree of social anomie, leaving individuals without the structures and expectations that are vital for a sense of identity.

The culture of self-sacrifice as the greatest form of heroism extolled by the Nazis was undoubtedly an important component in the suicides, especially amongst the military where it was considered an act of great patriotism and courage.[12] The propaganda at the time also encouraged the population to view self-sacrifice, to the point of death, as a demonstration of loyalty to the state. One propaganda article, written by Wilhelm Pleyer in March 1945, urges "to risk one's life does not merely mean to die, but also to really stand up for a cause ... and the desire to sacrifice one's personal existence" (Goeschel, p.154).

Suicides within the army were prevalent and often attributed to valor, but the reality for many soldiers may have been a mixture of fear of reprisals, the shame of defeat and what this meant for their future. A fictional account of suicide amongst soldiers at the front is given by the narrator of Starritt's novel, *We Germans*:

> There were suicides, more and more of them. Someone would go off to fetch water or rations and not come back. No one wanted to go looking, because you might find them slumped with their rifle in their lap. Also, if

their deaths were reported as suicides, their families wouldn't get a military pension. So we preferred not to look, and to assume that the Russians or the partisans had got them.

It was almost always under the trees. In the way that animals crawl under something when it's time to die, very few could bear to shoot themselves under the open sky.

But sometimes whole groups would shoot themselves together. Usually it would build up around a couple of men who'd served together for a long time, or even known each other before the war. I suppose each reminded the other that he had once been a man, not just a louse trying to evade the pinching fingers.

The group would go into the woods, drink bottles of stolen cognac, get sentimental, raise toasts until the cognac was finished and then all shoot themselves at once …

I saw these group suicides several times and never thought they were brave or honourable…

(Starritt, Loc. 565–74)

Amongst Hitler's top ranking officers, Goebbels fanned the flames of suicide most fervently, using the historic example of Frederick II's consideration of taking poison at a time of crisis as a model of heroic martyrdom. A clear message was broadcast that it is more honorable to kill oneself than accept defeat.[13] The Demmin Reverend Jacob Kronika wrote in his diary on 6th March 1945:

Wilhelm II promised us glorious times, but they didn't come. Hitler and Goebbels promise us large numbers of suicides and it's exactly what we get! That's what people are saying loud and clear in the air-raid shelter yesterday … The brunt of responsibility for this growing tendency to suicide falls on Dr Goebbels.

(Huber, p.79)

Suicide was not only licensed but encouraged by the state.

The sacralization of suicide was also linked directly to anxieties and fears of reprisals and life under the Allies. Fear of reprisals was an immediate widespread anxiety exacerbated by Nazi propaganda that spread horror stories of the brutality of the Russians.[14] As Jarausch comments:

Especially behind the Eastern Front, rumors of Russian atrocities spread like wildfire, fanned by a Nazi propaganda that tried to rally troops for a desperate defense through fear of revenge. When the Wehrmacht recaptured the village of Nemmersdorf in East Prussia, "our soldiers found the raped and mutilated bodies of women, children, and old men." They had been slaughtered indiscriminately. According to Ursula Mahlendorf,

Goebbels made the most of the massacre, screaming in a radio address, "This, my fellow countrymen, is what awaits you if you surrender! We will never surrender. You must fight to the last drop of blood!"

(Jarausch, p.179)

This propaganda made many people feel they had "no way out" after defeat; at the same time it also strengthened the population's sense that they were now the victims, suffering abuse from the hands of non-Germans.

Alongside this fear was a more pervasive existential fear of loss of identity and meaning, as signified by loss of a future. Goebbels eloquently describes this in his suicide note of 1st May 1945, clearly stating, "We have decided not to leave Berlin but to stay and end our life at our Fuhrer's side because to me life no longer holds value. I make this decision also on behalf of my children who are too young to offer their opinion but would surely come to the same conclusion if they were old enough."[15]

For many others, the vision they had held of belonging to a powerful and prosperous country that promised a rich future for them had shattered overnight. With nothing left, how could they go on? Peter Handke, in *A Sorrow Beyond Dreams*, describes his mother's restricted, featureless life before the war:

Personal life, if it had ever developed a character of its own, was depersonalised except for dream tatters swallowed up by the rites of religion, custom, and good manners; little remained of the human individual, and indeed, the word "individual" was known only in pejorative combinations ... The above-mentioned rites then functioned as a consolation. This consolation didn't address itself to you as a person; it simply swallowed you up, so that in the end you as an individual were content to be nothing, or at least nothing much.

(Handke, 2019, pp.40–1)

The advent of war suddenly opened up a new world for his mother, as for many young people at the time, one which was full of opportunities, the camaraderie of National Socialism and the feeling that she, along with others, was building a new life and a new country. She became an individual. With defeat, these opportunities and the vision of a future life had vanished and, while she survived and got along, even in the books she read, they were "never dreams of the future; in them she found everything she had missed and would never make good. Early in life she had dismissed all thought of a future" (Handke, p.52).

Handke is also describing the terrible loss and disillusionment experienced by Germans everywhere. Most survivors were able to build a new future but it is possible that for those who were not, they enacted their murderous rage against the Fuhrer by killing themselves. In this way, Hitler's followers could maintain their idealization of their leader and protect the ideals they had espoused while, unconsciously, killing the leader who had duped them.

Finally, there is the supposition that the mass suicides committed at the end of the war were committed by guilt. *Life Magazine* reported on 14th May 1945 that: "In the last days of the war the overwhelming realization of utter defeat was too much for many Germans. Stripped of the bayonets and bombast which had given them power, they could not face a reckoning with either their conquerors or their consciences." This supposition assumes that the German population as a whole, facing defeat and awareness of the crimes that had been committed in the name of the Reich, had guilty consciences that led many to commit suicide.

There is in fact scant evidence that clearly points to guilt being an important feature of the mass suicides. Amongst the top Nazi leaders who committed suicide, including those who were tried and convicted at Nuremburg, admission of guilt was notably absent. Some individual accounts come close to an admission of guilt but other factors, such as fear of retribution, are also likely. One navy officer, on being told the war had ended, decided to shoot himself, explaining, "Given my conduct throughout the war, I had no hope of survival, and felt that only death could mask my shame" (Huber, p.106). It is not clear what the officer means when he writes he had "no hope of survival", perhaps he was frightened of reprisals or punishment, but his feeling of shame is also ambiguous. Shame is not guilt and suggests the officer may have been more frightened of being exposed to have done something wrong or even to have failed to win the war; it does not indicate guilt for wrongdoing. A student commented, "A friend of mine killed herself when she heard the truth … and she wasn't the only one" (Huber, p.105). Here again, the friend may have killed herself from shame but it may also have been from the shock of betrayal and the sudden collapse of a world she had trusted. Such accounts do not confirm guilt. But for the Allies arriving as victors it was particularly difficult, with knowledge of the extermination camps and other wartime atrocities, to comprehend how Germans, struggling to adapt to and survive their ruined circumstances, could not possibly feel guilty.

Alongside the shock of defeat, the Germans had to face the hatred of the Allies. The narrator in *We Germans*, expresses this clearly:

> We Germans (had) gone from being the new masters of Europe to being the hated Germans, the fucking Germans, what the Russians called "the accursed Germany". And being hated while you're winning is one thing; it's quite another to be hated while you lose.
>
> (Starritt, Loc. 520–9)

This collective hatred amongst the Allies served to exacerbate the view of the Germans as victims, not as perpetrators.

What is clear from these different explanations and from diaries and suicide notes from the time is that the popular narratives centred around the themes of loyalty to the Fuhrer, fear of reprisals, the shame of defeat, and overwhelming loss (i.e. the loss of a future). The narratives are necessarily fluid and not mutually exclusive but they suggest that those who committed suicide had largely supported the regime. What is missing are narratives that might have come from those who objected to or resisted the regime – unless these would be under the category of fear of reprisals. The absence of this kind of narrative raises the important question as to why, especially amongst those who objected to the regime, did they not kill themselves because they felt guilty, for example, for failing to be more active in their resistance? Is it possible for those who may have felt guilty that the end of the war was welcome as it relieved them of some guilt? Or is it possible that those who had not supported the regime were less vulnerable to suicide?

The Imposition of Guilt

When people, either individually or as part of a group, are found guilty of committing a crime, it does not necessarily follow that they feel guilty, even though they may acknowledge that a crime has been committed. In Germany, some, like Renate Finckh, experienced "remorse and shame". These affects seem to have more to do with being connected to a group found guilty (in the sense of being culpable) of inflicting harm; they are not the same as feeling guilt. Although there is a great deal of evidence that much of the German population was aware of the atrocities being committed[16] and the excuse of ignorance is only partly true, it is important to recognize that the population was not a homogenous mass but held different roles and perspectives in relation to what they were aware of and what they actually witnessed. Finckh recalls witnessing the attacks on Jews and her father's admonition, "But you and I, we're nothing to do with all that, do you hear!" (Huber, p.200). Psychological techniques of denial, dissociation, distancing and repression enabled ordinary citizens and those working directly for the regime to separate their own internal beliefs from their external reality; in this way, the psychosis of war and its consequences could be protected against. There were also increasingly harsh penalties for challenging the regime and its actions that effectively silenced many witnesses. Under a fascist government that exacted compliance if not active allegiance, there is no place for individual protest except through underground methods. Given this, saying that the population should feel guilty for crimes licensed by the state conflates any distinction between the individual and the state. Similarly, within democratic systems of government that allow citizens to protest, while they are responsible for their government, this does not make them guilty of their government's misdeeds.[17]

The conflation between the individual and the state indicates a confusion in the distinction between responsibility and guilt. The philosopher, Susan Neiman, in her recent book, *Learning from the Germans*, attempts to explore this distinction and ends up questioning whether responsibility and guilt can be separated. It is understandable that this is her conclusion because it is apparent in her thinking that there is no question as to whether or not Germans are and feel guilty – they must be so even if they don't acknowledge it. Neiman refers to The Group Experiment conducted by Theodor Adorno and Max Horkheimer in 1949. A group of eighteen hundred people, from all walks of life, were invited to speak about German guilt. Neiman comments:

> Though the participants represented a large variety of occupations and education, their language and historical references suggest fairly high capacities for reflection. They just didn't use them. None expressed a desire to return to the good old days of the Third Reich. Perhaps they were wary of doing so in front of the experimenters facilitating the discussions, but whatever memories they had of peace, prosperity, and pride in the '30s were battered by what followed. Stalingrad at the front and bombed-out cities at home produced shock and shame that were amply clear in 1950. The shame, however, had no moral component. Nearly every participant in the Group Experiment denied any suggestion of guilt ... Pointing to other nations' sins, with a special focus on America, was a favored defense against recognizing their own.
>
> (Neiman, 2019, pp.50–1)

Neiman's stance of moral superiority and self-righteousness is clear. She describes the group as having "fairly high capacities for reflection" and yet "They just didn't use them". She continues to point out that while the group expressed shame about the inhumanity of the Nazi regime, they "denied any suggestion of guilt". Adorno and his team, for example, tried to understand the denial of guilt in the group by psychoanalytic concepts of paranoia and infantile narcissism. Neiman comments about the team: "They do not seek to analyse why one woman responded to moral catastrophe in the *right way*, with a knowledge of sin and a sense of guilt that demanded expiation, cost what it may for herself and her children" (Neiman, p.52). It is impossible for Neiman – or Adorno and his team – to believe that the group did not feel guilt. Even when members of the group accepted the crimes that had been committed by the Germans, they argued other nations had committed worse. Neiman assumes that there was something wrong with the group, not with the assumptions made by Adorno and his colleagues, or herself for that matter. She is also clear that the shame expressed "had no moral component". By this, Neiman suggests that shame has no moral component because it does not recognize harm to others. However, the definition of shame is "a painful feeling of humiliation or distress caused by the consciousness of wrong or foolish behavior," "a regrettable or unfortunate situation or action." (OED) The experience of shame is founded on a sense of morality, of what is right and wrong. However, what is shameful is linked to behavior that is antithetical to the individual and culturally ideal image we have of ourselves. It does not necessarily encompass our behavior towards others and the feelings of guilt that may ensue from this (See Chapter Four).

Neiman is not alone in her assumption that Germans "must" be and feel guilty, just as she argues that the offspring of Southern families "must" similarly be and feel guilty about slavery. However, in this assumption, she also implies that the Germans and the American southerners have committed worse crimes than other nations or groups. This is precisely what Neiman accuses the German participants of doing. In the case of the Germans, we can imagine that they may well have been sick of being accused of being guilty and may have been reacting defensively or have needed to minimize the extremity of crimes committed in comparison with others in order not to be singled out as evil. In Neiman's case, however, her assignation of guilt across a population comes across as self-righteous demonization.

Neiman asserts that a group becomes moral and morally acceptable when they acknowledge guilt on the basis that "our past will haunt us if we do not face it down" (Neiman, p.39). It is unclear, however, what is meant by "acknowledging guilt" and what is meant by "facing it down". Groups need to be able to acknowledge the harm they have caused others as a way of maintaining social morality and validating the group's reality. Acknowledging what the group has done – whether for bad or for good – is also vital in establishing a group's self-agency. This applies to admitting culpability for harm; but admitting culpability is not the same as being or feeling guilty.

Psychoanalysts are also amongst those who have made the assumption that the German population must experience collective guilt. Hella Ehlers asks:

> What were the effects of the severe blow Germans of this generation received to their inflated and aggressive form of narcissism when the Nazi regime was finally defeated and its power base destroyed? What happened to this pathology under the impact of this trauma? Have Germans of this generation really understood the state of mind they were in, which drove and seduced them into colluding with Nazi propaganda, making Hitler their *Fuhrer* and his ideals their own? After all, reading *Mein Kampf* would have found it staring them in the face ... The more acute question facing us today is how this has affected the generation of their children and how they can come to terms with their experience. What, for example, are the effects on them of a psychotic part in their parents' personality ... which was involved in the Nazi experience of the past and was never subsequently integrated into the healthier part of the personality?
>
> (Ehlers & Crick, 1994, pp.16–7)

We have some answers to Ehlers's question about the impact of the fall of the regime in the mass suicides alone, in those who felt their future had vanished, in those who had felt deceived by Hitler's vision and in the ways in which

East and West Germans created new narratives of the future. Ehlers writes in 1994, and there is now much more research material available regarding postwar Germany and reconstruction, but it is clear that Ehlers has little conception of how large groups can be seduced and indoctrinated, how they can follow charismatic leaders despite their policies and actions, and how important a belief in a powerful future can be when a country has suffered from defeat and humiliation in the past.[18] Ehlers also makes the mistake of treating the Nazi generation and their offspring as one entity. Perhaps her description of the "psychotic parts of (the) personality" of the parents applies to those officers who served within the regime and who committed atrocities, but even this is a form of mass labelling in which evil actions are explained by madness. For the ordinary German citizen, this description may have little relevance and even less so for the next generation. Another common assumption is that the silence of parents about their Nazi past came from their feelings of unspeakable guilt which were then transmitted to their children. It is possible to imagine that many of these children may have lived with depressed parents and have suffered from neurotic guilt, feeling responsible for their parents' depression, taking on omnipotent responsibility for causing them pain while feeling helpless themselves. Silent parents may have felt depressed because of losing the war, or because of how the regime had destroyed their lives, but, here again, this does not mean their silence was due to guilt.

Alexander and Margarette Mitscherlich produced the famous psychoanalytic postwar study of guilt in Germany, entitled, *The Inability to Mourn* (1975). As with Adorno's experiment, the Mitscherlichs noted the striking absence of guilt in the German population following the end of the war. They write:

> Declared Nazis virtually never appeared: insofar as they had remained such, they obviously managed very well by continuing their idealizations, projections, and resentments; possibly by associating themselves with extreme right-wing groups. This small group of people did not deny the crimes of the Third Reich; they merely denied that such acts were criminal. In view of the meagerness of any outward signs of an inner burden that could not be managed by normal means, one might have gathered that Germany had never been Nazi and that in 1945 it had at most lost a group of Nazi, that is to say foreign, occupiers.
>
> (Mitscherlich & Mitscherlich, p.32)

They argued that once these defense mechanisms broke down:

> The ego is then faced with a new task; that of coping with the guilt accumulated during the phase of collective delusion. This can be done either by a remorseful realization and acceptance of what has happened, or by resorting to defense mechanisms against the menacing reality, such as all of us used in childhood against the fear of punishment ... It should

be noted, moreover, that defense against a collectively incurred guilt is easy when it, too, is carried out collectively, since the degree of guilt is then determined by universal consensus. Normally, a guilt-laden individual is isolated from society; but in a group he does not endure this fate, being merely a sinner among sinners.

(Ibid., p.33)

The Mitscherlichs analysis of collective guilt and its denial is in line with psychoanalytic theory based on the study of individual patients. But certain questions arise in the case of collective behavior. The Mitscherlichs refer to the period under the Reich as "the phase of collective delusion" and assume that, once this delusion is broken, the population will have to face the crimes that were committed, making a further assumption that feelings of guilt will necessarily accompany this. However, the Mitscherlichs also accede that the consequences of wrongdoing by a group are not the same as in the case of an individual; for a start there is no isolation from the group. They also assert the psychoanalytic principle that the process of mourning cannot occur without an acknowledgement and acceptance of guilt. They do not question whether in fact there is such a thing as collective guilt, or collective mourning for that matter (See Chapter Seven).[19]

Prior to reunification, the West Germans have been extolled for their Holocaust memorials and public admissions of guilt, most notably signified by Willy Brandt's gesture of penance as he knelt in front of the *Warsaw Ghetto Uprising* memorial in 1970. These collective admissions of wrongdoing have an impact on collective awareness, certainly if nothing else, to establish and memorialize historical events in the collective psyche. But there is a difference between these signifiers and what the collective *feels*. Furthermore, while we might well wonder whether the generation of the Reich, especially those actively engaged in committing atrocities, may have felt guilt about the destructiveness of the regime, it is by no means clear that this was a collective feeling. As noted, most Germans were primarily concerned about their material survival and had their own losses to mourn. After defeat and the vilification of the Reich, grief about the loss of Hitler and the Nazi ideal was all but censored publicly, leaving an unspoken bitterness amongst many Nazi supporters. From this perspective, other losses seemed secondary.

Michael Gorra, in his review of Neiman's *Learning from the Germans*, describes coming across a plaque in the Bavarian city of Landshut declaring, "In 1939 18.7 million Germans lived in territories from which they would be expelled – and it went on to say that between 1944 and 1946 they were thrown out, displaced, murdered, or went missing. Twelve million, the plaque added, would live to arrive in Germany ..."

Millions of ethnic Germans – Volksdeutsche – had been expelled from Eastern Europe in the aftermath of WWII and resettled in the West. In their new homes they formed fraternal societies and insisted they had a claim to their old ones; their sense of aggrieved nostalgia played a major part in the conservative politics of Bavaria in particular. We suffered too, the Landshut memorial claims, we too were victims ... (T)he mood in West Germany in the first decades after the war was closer to that of the Landshut memorial than one likes to remember.

(Gorra, 2019, p.11)

For the next generation, the question of collective guilt becomes even more problematic as they are the inheritors of their parents' history. Children of high-ranking Nazi officers or those who were known to have committed war crimes had to come to terms with what their parents had done and the opprobrium of the world that highlighted their parents' crimes. There were also the so-called "atonement Germans", such as the Mitscherlichs, who claimed that the German population was suffering from guilt and needed to acknowledge this to form a healthy nation.

This societal pressure has created a complex burden for those born after the war, many of whom felt they were being asked to carry the guilt and shame of deeds they had not done and had no influence on. For those who grew up under a cloud of guilt, personal unhappiness could be subsumed (and confused) with the crimes their parents had committed and wellbeing could be tinged with guilt. Iris Hanika's novel, *The Bureau of Past Management*, describes the conflict about what it means to be German. The narrator, a Holocaust archivist, reflects on his experience, "He learned to differentiate the Germany he lived in from the era he worked on ... He had taken a long time to admit he liked his country. Once it would have seemed like a betrayal" (Hanika, 2021, p.14).

Being identified with and identifying oneself as German results in an emotional impasse; assuming false guilt unconsciously gives "the other", i.e. members of the formerly attacked groups, the power to exonerate the guilty. In this way, the guilty party is dependent on "the other" to feel that they are not "bad" anymore. However, because this process is based on a false premise, it does not ring true. As a result, many Germans today bear a mixture of pity and contempt, largely unspoken, for those who profess guilt on behalf of the perpetrator generation (Scholz, 2020, pp.86–7). Apologies for someone else's crimes are not only misplaced but presumptuous.

The taking on of guilt for others assumes an omnipotent responsibility for the past and at the same time exonerates contemporary Germans who are not "like that". This self-righteous position reflects the attitudes of the Allies after the war that carries on to this day, of pointing to Nazi Germany as the historic epicenter of evil, enabling other countries conveniently to deny their own crimes and to locate them elsewhere. Guilt, like evil, is then distanced from all of us and is something that happens and is done by "others", not us.

Arendt is clear about the philosophical and social limits of guilt and contemptuous of the guilt expressed by those who were not involved in the war. She writes:

… if young people in Germany, too young to have done anything at all, feel guilty they are either wrong, confused, or they are playing at intellectual games. There is no such thing as collective guilt or collective innocence; guilt and innocence make sense only if applied to individuals.

(Arendt, 2003, p,29)

By asserting that innocence is equally something that belongs to individuals and not the collective, Arendt is also emphasizing the danger of this kind of binary splitting whereby one group is deemed "bad", enabling one's own group to remain "pure" and "good". This was precisely the kind of projection and splitting that Hitler promoted under the Reich.

Viktor Frankl, in his speech in 1988 marking Austria's annexation by Germany in 1938, echoes Arendt's views. Frankl warns:

I ask you not to expect a single word of hatred from me. Who should I hate? I know only the victims but I do not know the perpetrators, at least I do not know them personally and to blame somebody not personally but collectively, is something I strictly reject. Collective guilt does not exist! … I believe that to collectively blame the men and women in Austria who are today between 0 and 50 years old is a crime and madness or let me formulate it in a psychiatric manner: It would be a crime if it wasn't a case of madness and in addition a relapse into the National Socialists' ideology of "clan liability". Let this be said to those who believe they are justified in saying that you have to feel guilty or even ashamed of something you did not do yourself or did not even refrain from doing yourself but something the parents or even the grandparents burdened their conscience with. And I think I am sure that the victims of former collective persecution should and will be the first to agree with me, unless their intention is to drive the youth of today into the hands of the old Nazis or the Neo-Nazis.

Critics of Frankl accuse him of giving license to nations not to take responsibility for their past because they are not guilty. Here again is the conflation of acknowledgement of past events with how the collective *ought* to feel about it. Frankl, like Arendt, is wary of the demonization of any group because of what it led to under the Reich. His words indicate that taking on the mantle of collective guilt, rather than leading to a healthier society, may paradoxically maintain the madness of "clan liability". Blaming the Germans with the expectation that they should acknowledge their guilt (versus culpability) can be understood as an effort to re-establish social order and a clear delineation between good and evil. According to Judeo-Christian beliefs as well as psychoanalytic theory, the process of collective mourning and reparation could then take place – but did they?

Reparation and Racial Hatred

Regardless of whether we consider collective guilt to be a viable concept, the racial hatred that was the at the heart of Hitler's regime has not disappeared; it continues, evident today in the rise of neo-fascist, alt-right political groups, despite attempts on the part of the German government to suppress it. Racial hatred in both East and West Germany is nothing new and notably re-emerged in Germany after reunification.[20] Over a period of three days in August 1992, the first xenophobic attack took place in East Germany (in Rostock-Lichtenhagen) in which a tower block, inhabited by Vietnamese workers (employed during the GDR), was set on fire while a crowd of about 3000 people applauded. The police did not appear until it was too late. Much of the frustration and anger against the new regime of reunification, and the loss and disappointment that followed, was displaced onto foreigners. By attacking foreign and weaker groups, the former East Germans could feel empowered, identifying with their oppressors in a repeated cycle of abuse and humiliation.[21]

Racist attacks were not, however, restricted to the East; fire attacks on houses inhabited by foreigners also occurred in the West. The Iron Curtain had established clear divides between external and internal worlds and had created a clear social order. When the Iron Curtain came down and identities on both sides were threatened, the conflicts both within and outside the two worlds surfaced.

Racial hatred is not endemic or in any way specific to Germany, as we are witnessing around the world today. However, there is an expectation in post-genocidal countries, such as Germany, Rwanda, Serbia and elsewhere, that recognition of the atrocities committed and processes of reconciliation, guilt and forgiveness will prevent future outbreaks of hatred. What we are seeing instead is that hatred of the "other", either lying dormant or repressed for a time, tends to rear its head and emerge when large groups become anxious about their identity and survival. We have seen this happen most recently in the United States with racist attacks on black Americans, despite years of protest and struggle to create racial equality. We are left with doubts about the nature of collective guilt, whether feelings of guilt can be attributed to large groups at all, and whether processes of mourning and reparation are concepts that fundamentally change political dynamics as opposed to ritual performances that establish a redistribution of power and temporary peace. Old tribal hatreds continue to live within us all and, like the return of the repressed, are hard to extinguish.

Notes

1 Amongst the Western Allies, the Americans adopted a particularly punitive attitude towards the Germans, encouraging American soldiers to view Germans as the "enemy". Prohibitions on fraternization were notable, as outlined in the G-3 US Army handbook, instructing soldiers to behave with "cool hostility and distaste…" and to make it "clear to the Germans that they are responsible for the Second World War and will not be forgiven their terrible oppression of other peoples under

German rule." (quoted in Jahner, H. (2019). *Aftermath: Life in the Fallout of the Third Reich, 1945–1955*. London: W.H. Allen, p.244)

2 There is a growing body of literature written by Germans who were cognizant of what was going on within the Reich and opposed to Hitler. See, for example, Haffner, S., *Defying Hitler: A Memoir*, Phoenix, 2011 and *My Opposition: The Diary of Friedrich Kellner, A German against the Third Reich*, ed. S. Kellner, Cambridge: Cambridge University Press, 2018.

3 Berlin, with its predominantly female population at the end of the war, was known for the *Trummerfrauen*, the "rubble women". At the height of the clearance work, 26,000 women were engaged in hard labor as compared to 9,000 men. (Jahner, *Aftermath*, p.20.)

4 If the West Germans had not had contact with the outside world it is arguable that they might not have had any reason to assume social guilt.

5 In West Germany in the 1950s approximately three quarters of the judges and lawyers who had served under the Reich had been reinstated to their former positions. The plea of "following orders", in this case upholding the law of the land, was a strong mitigating factor that did not carry such weight in East Germany.

6 In his book on the Stasi, Koehler writes, "To ensure that the people would become and remain submissive, East German communist leaders saturated their realm with more spies than had any other totalitarian government in recent history." (Stasi)

7 The recognition in 1948 of genocide as a war crime and the subsequent establishment of the International Criminal Court in 2001 to adjudicate war crimes under international law provided an ultimate witness to atrocities committed under certain national regimes. It is striking that these legal processes were inevitably aimed at individual perpetrators and could not, as such, hold nations accountable for collective crimes.

8 Germany's postwar pacifism is often attributed to the recognition and acceptance of the criminality of the Reich. While many Germans felt tainted by their experience of war, this does not suggest evidence of guilt.

9 Jahner comments that those former Nazis who had felt betrayed were able to adopt democracy and denazification through the process of "self-victimization" that absolved them of "any obligation they might otherwise have felt to engage with the Nazi crimes committed in their name. Jahner argues that the "communicative silencing" of the past, as described by the philosopher Jermann Lubbe, "made it possible for tens of millions of still devoted Nazis to integrate themselves into a society that had made a consensus out of anti-fascism, in terms of both its constitution and self-image." (Jahner, *Aftermath*, pp.316–7)

10 After the Japanese defeat in Okinawa in June 1945, the population was similarly encouraged to kill themselves through fear of reprisals and loyalty to the Emperor. The narrator of *Fracture*, a novel by Andres Neuman, states: "I was very shocked by the stories about Okinawa. When they lost that last battle, the army convinced civilians that the enemy would torture them and massacre their families if they didn't take their own lives. They say that many people got their friends to kill them. Others lay in a circle around the grenades they had been given. Whole families committed suicide together. The father was usually the one who removed the pin. For the few who didn't kill themselves, falling into enemy hands proved less deadly than obeying their own army. That must have felt very odd. The survivors ended up strangely grateful to the invaders for having spared them. A Japanese-style Stockholm syndrome." Neuman, A. (2020). *Fracture*. London: Granta Books. Loc 3299.

11 The suicide figures in Berlin during 1945 rose to more than 7,000.

12 Jarausch notes: "Unable to bear the shame of loss, some officers committed suicide rather than be captured. Many ordinary soldiers, such as Karl Hartel, were depressed, because 'at the bitter end we lost the war and everything such as home, property, and the claim to justice before history.' By contrast, Hans Queiser 'was neither dejected nor desperate,' because no 'Germany' and certainly no Fuhrer remained in his head. Only the will to get through what would now follow and then to go home."(Jarausch, p.143)

13 On 12th April 1945, during the last concert of the Berlin Philharmonic, Hitler Youth handed out cyanide pills to the audience.

14 Anthony Beevor, the historian, describes the Russian takeover of East Prussia, Pomerania and Silesia as the scene for the "greatest phenomenon of mass rape in history." Approximately 1.4 million women were raped.

15 Goebbels and his wife poisoned themselves and their five children.

16 See especially Horowitz, G.J. (1990), *In the Shadow of Death: Living Outside the Gates of Mauthausen*, Oxford: Macmillan; Fulbrook, M, (2012), *A Small Town Near Auschwitz: Ordinary Nazis and the Holocaust*, Oxford: Oxford University Press; and Kellner, R.S. (ed.) (2018), *My Opposition: The Diary of Friedrich Kellner – A German Against the Third Reich*, Cambridge: Cambridge University Press.

17 Trump's family separation immigration policy, enacted from April through June 2018, is a case in point in which there was clear disagreement and protest that was largely disregarded by the government. Does this mean that the American population is guilty of inflicting this harm on immigrant families? On a larger scale, the Vietnam War was extremely contentious within the US and, while the US has been widely criticized for its involvement in the war, its population is not held to be guilty of the atrocities and loss of lives incurred.

18 For an analysis of this process, see Janine Chasseguet-Smirgel's essay, "The Ego Ideal and the Group", in *The Ego Ideal* (1985), London: Free Association Books.

19 Following the Rwandan genocide, the President, Paul Kagame, invited Dr Colin Murray Parkes, a British psychiatrist who pioneered work on mourning, to assist his country in mourning. Years later, Dr Murray Parkes expressed doubts about whether large groups could mourn as he felt his work in Rwanda had failed to achieve this, as evident by the continuing deep-seated animosity between the Hutus and the Tutsis that is expected to resurface upon Kagame's stepping down from the presidency. (Personal communication from Dr Murray Parkes)

20 The influx of German immigrants from Eastern Europe, referred to as "Zuzugler", into both East and West Germany was widely resented by the local population who considered the incomers as foreigners and not belonging. Being German was no exemption from persecution against immigrants. (See Jahner, *Aftermath*, p.67)

21 In the East there was a long history of racism against the Slavs, referred to as the "Untermensch", the not human. The hatred of the Slavs accounts to some extent for the terrible war crimes committed in the Eastern bloc countries and Russia, most notably in the siege of Leningrad. Fear of Russian/Slavic reprisals was particularly acute amongst East Germans.

References

Arendt, H. (2003). *Responsibility and Judgment*. New York: Schocken Books.

Ehlers, H. and Crick, J. (1994). *The Trauma of the Past: Remembering and Working Through*. London: Goethe Institute.

Frankl, Viktor (1988). *Speech marking Austria's annexation by Germany in 1938*.

Fulbrook, M. (2018). *Reckonings: Legacies of Nazi Persecution and the Quest for Justice*. Oxford: Oxford University Press.

Goeschel, C. (2009). *Suicide in Nazi Germany.* Oxford: Oxford University Press.

Gorra, M. (7 November 2019). "A Heritage of Evil." *New York Review of Books.*

Handke, P. (2019). *A Sorrow Beyond Dreams.* London: Pushkin Press.

Hanika, I. (2021). *The Bureau of Past Management.* London: V&Q Books.

Heise, V. (2020). *Berlin 1945.* London: BBC Documentary.

Huber, F. (2019). *Promise Me You'll Shoot Yourself: The Downfall of Ordinary Germans in 1945.* London: Penguin Random House UK.

Jarausch, K.H. (2018). *Broken Lives: How Ordinary Germans Experienced the 20th Century.* Princeton: Princeton University Press.

Koehler, J.O. (1999). *Stasi: The Untold Story of The East German Secret Police.* Oxford: Westview Press.

Mitscherlich, A. and Mitscherlich, M. (1975). *The Inability to Mourn: Principles of Collective Behavior.* New York: Grove Press, Inc.

Neiman, S. (2019). *Learning from the Germans: Confronting Race and the Memory of Evil.* London: Allen Lane.

Scholz, R. (2020). "The German 'Welcoming Culture': some thoughts about its psychodynamics." In: Zajenkowska, A. and Levin, U. (eds) (2020). *A Psychoanalytic and Socio-Cultural Exploration of a Continent.* London: Routledge, pp. 85–98.

Starritt, A. (2020). *We Germans.* London: John Murray.

Chapter 4

Guilt and Shame

> I'm ashamed of my family, of what they've done to others and to me. It makes me feel dirty and exposed. Guilt is a very different feeling – that's for the things I can control.
>
> (Kerry, abused)

Introduction

At the end of World War Two, a young German woman, Ingeborg Bachmann, records in her diary being interrogated about her membership in an organization, the "Bund Deutscher Mädel", that was part of the Hitler Youth movement. She admits that "I blushed bright red and I was so desperate I went even redder", despite the fact that she had replied truthfully that she had not attended any gatherings or meetings since she was fourteen. Hans Holler, in his Afterword to Ingeborg's *War Diary*, comments:

> She simply couldn't understand "why you blush and tremble when you're telling the truth" – as if the psychosomatic reaction indicates uncertainty and shame which lies outside the Yes or No of her answers. However inappropriate this body language might seem, as a writer Bachmann took it seriously. In her literary work as well as in her theoretical essays she constantly examined the connection between "politics and physiology", as if there was something, in the "completely incomprehensible realm", that suggested a deeper level of reality.
>
> (Bachmann, 2018, p.78)

At the age of eighteen, Bachmann was clear about her hatred of Nazism and the war; she was also clear that she was not blushing out of guilt, she had told the truth and did not feel responsible for the devastation the Third Reich had left behind. And yet her blushing exposed a more unconscious connection to what had happened, one in which she was inextricably implicated through shame.

DOI: 10.4324/9781003379980-5

Guilt and shame are often used interchangeably despite their distinct and different meanings. This confusion may arise because each confers a state of contamination that affects not only individuals but groups; their stigma can then be interpreted as a mark of responsibility, as having broken a moral or social code. This confusion, particularly when groups are accused of collective guilt for their misdeeds, allows us not only to point the finger of blame at someone or some group but it creates an illusion that there is always someone responsible and, along with this, that we are in control of our fate. This is not to say that people and groups are not responsible for the crimes they commit, but that the most important distinguishing feature of guilt is that it is the result of an action within our control and responsibility, whereas shame is the result of that which is beyond our control. Both guilt and shame result from the breaking of social norms or rules that places the individual or group as "other". But there are significant psychological and social differences between the two and the status they confer.

Carlo Ginzburg, in his essay, "The Bond of Shame", vividly describes the experience, "Shame is definitely not a matter of choice: it falls upon us, invading us – our bodies, our feelings, our thoughts – as a sudden illness." (Ginzburg, 2019, p.35) The description of shame as something that "falls upon us" applies to both victims and perpetrators. For victims, the erasure of human dignity imposes personal shame just as they are sullied socially.[1] Perpetrators also experience shame in actions that abnegate the self. Guilt, on the other hand, arises out of choice, even if it is the choice of failing to act; it is a violation of one's conscience that is specific to an act that has harmful consequences for an "other". If no harm is perceived, there is nothing to feel guilty about. Shame, as Ginzburg writes, "falls upon us" and is an aversive reaction to being seen by others as inferior, weak, or in the wrong. Shame is a loss of face, it is not concerned with wrong doing so much as wrong being, as we see in Bachmann's blush. The primary concept that steers us in distinguishing between guilt and shame is free will or the idea of self-agency. Guilt derives from an action or a failure to act that results in harm towards someone else and, as an act, expresses self-agency; shame is the absence of self-agency.

Definitions and Distinctions

Original Sin

In Judeo-Christian tradition, we can thank Adam and Eve, and perhaps most importantly, the Serpent in the Garden of Eden for our human plight. Mortality, pain, the need to work to survive, guilt and shame were all incurred as punishment for eating the fruit from the Tree of Knowledge. The Serpent persuades Eve that eating the forbidden apple[2] will not result in death but will give Eve and her partner, Adam, the knowledge of good and evil that only

God has. Ironically, the temptation to acquire god-like omniscience in relation to good and evil is what gives mankind the free will to choose between
them. But free will only arises with the loss of innocence, precipitated by the
Serpent, God's trickster who deceives Adam and Eve into believing that they
are not in fact committing a crime. Eating the apple is the only forbidden act
in the Garden of Eden that God has laid out – by disobeying God, Adam
and Eve challenge God's omnipotence and enter a new reality in which good
and evil co-exist and affect every action of man. The choice to disobey
also brings with it a new self-consciousness whereby man sees himself as
human and, as such, as having both the ability to choose and the inability
to control all his actions. This is the root of free will and at the same time
our awareness of our capacity for evil, for a destructiveness that originates
in our defiance of God.

The crime of "original sin" is inexorably accompanied by man's first
experience of shame. Man's nakedness, his human weakness, becomes shameful.
Adam responds to the call of God after the Fall,

> I heard thy voice in the garden, and I was afraid, because I was naked;
> and I hid myself. And he (i.e. God) said, Who told thee that thou was
> naked? Hast thou eaten of the tree whereof I commanded thee, that thou
> shouldest not eat?
>
> (Bible, Gen. 3, pp.10–1)

Adam now needs to hide his nakedness from God's eyes in shame; a shame
that did not exist prior to eating the apple. But shame is not the simple outcome of breaking God's law; it signifies an awareness of human vulnerability
that comes from our inability to control our bodily functions and our most
primitive impulses. Shame derives from being shown up, from losing face
before God. Adam and Eve's innocent status before God has been tarnished
in their defiance of God's will. Eating the apple was an act of free will, the
step that marked man's independence from God. At the same time eating the
apple brought into consciousness that our impulses or instinctual responses
are not always within our control. This is ultimately what led to Adam and
Eve's downfall and their shame. It was this act of free will that gave Adam
and Eve responsibility over their actions and the knowledge of good and evil;
at the same time in failing God, Adam and Eve experienced shame in their
failure to control their impulses. The knowledge of man's vulnerability, of not
being able to control his impulses, is both God's gift to man and His curse.

The philosopher, J. David Velleman, elucidates the significance played by
the sudden intertwined awareness of involuntary control and will experienced
by Adam and Eve in the Fall.

> Having their eyes opened would not in itself have caused Adam and Eve
> to lose voluntary control that they previously possessed. But a slightly

different alteration could indeed have been brought about by the acquisition of knowledge and, in particular, by that knowledge of good and evil which Adam and Eve acquired in eating from the tree. For suppose ... that this episode taught them about good and evil by teaching them about the possibility of disobeying God and their God-given instincts. In that case, they must previously have been unaware that disobeying God and Nature was a possibility, and so they must have been in no position to disobey. They would have slavishly done as God and their instincts demanded, because of being unaware that they might do otherwise. And if they slavishly obeyed these demands, without a thought of doing otherwise, then their free will would have been no more than a dormant capacity, which they wouldn't exercise until they discovered the possibility of alternatives on which to exercise it. That discovery, imparted by the serpent, would thus have activated the hitherto dormant human will, thereby making it fully effective for the first time since the Creation. On this interpretation, the reason why Adam and Eve weren't ashamed of their nakedness at first is not that their anatomy was perfectly subordinate to the will but rather that they didn't have an effective will to which their anatomy could be insubordinate. In acquiring the idea of making choices contrary to the demands of their instincts, however, they would have gained, not only the effective capacity to make those choices, but also the realization that their bodies might obey their instincts instead, thus proving insubordinate to their newly activated will. Hence the knowledge that would have activated their will could also have opened their eyes to the possibility of that bodily recalcitrance which Augustine identifies as the occasion of their shame.

(Velleman, 2001, p.34)

Velleman argues that shame, in the context of the story of the Fall, comes about when we are in a situation that exposes the fact that our bodily instincts are insubordinate to our will. The Fall represents the caesura that is opened between our natural instincts (however we describe these) and human will. Paradoxically, it is this caesura that introduces the possibility of free will. This is strikingly illustrated in child development. For the toddler, discovering he can say "no" is the point at which he first exercises conscious control or will. It is also at this time that children first visibly experience shame, when they are aware of not being able to control themselves or the objects around them despite their intentions. In asserting his will, the child immediately becomes aware of his authority in the world and how he is perceived by others – he establishes a social face.[3] This is also what makes him vulnerable to failure, to loss of control, to loss of face and, hence, to shame. Without a "face", i.e. without self-agency, there is no face to lose. The ability to say "no" and to exercise free will leads to a self-consciousness that would not have previously existed for Adam and Eve nor would this have been a necessary function to their existence.

Shame and the Ideal Self

The Fall from the Garden of Eden has been likened to the infant's dawning awareness of his lack of omnipotence as he becomes aware of his separateness from the breast. This narcissistic rupture creates recognition of the other and the beginnings of relatedness that can produce and inflict pain and pleasure with ensuing feelings of guilt or satisfaction. It also establishes the beginnings of how the infant sees himself through the interactive feedback loop of the mother's perception and experience her baby. When the infant feels at one with the mother without frustration or self-consciousness (i.e. self-judgement), this can be likened, certainly in our fantasy, to Adam and Eve's experience in the Garden of Eden; the breast is always at hand, the weather always the right temperature and paradise is there to fulfill one's every wish seamlessly and effortlessly. Like the infant's sudden loss of the breast, Adam and Eve's expulsion from Eden must have felt like a bumpy and shocking landing on a concrete runway. Coming down to earth and harsh reality would certainly make them painfully aware of their vulnerability and their dependence on each other for their survival. Stripped of their sense of entitlement, we can well imagine the shame Adam and Eve may have felt on arrival as their narcissism had suffered quite a blow.

Shame is a direct product of narcissism, both in relation to individuals and groups, as it is fundamentally linked to how we are seen by others and to our image of our ideal self, i.e. who is the person I aspire to be in the world so that I can be loved and admired. The ideal self is like a North Star to the ego, guiding it in its actions and enabling it to navigate the conflicts and opportunities life presents. This image of our ideal self starts forming during infancy when we discover what emotional effect we have on others and learn what behavior and attitudes are praised and what are not. Our super-ego acts as a kind of mediator and judge, holding the ego to task against the image of our ideal ego. When there is a disjunction between the ego ideal and the ego, the ego is put to shame. The classic example of one of our first experiences of shame is the toddler who is being potty-trained and soils himself by mistake. The failure to control bodily functions which has formed part of the ego ideal is exposed for all to see and creates a narcissistic hurt that affects self-esteem and is intrinsically related to how the self is seen by others. This connection between the ego ideal and the environment that shapes it establishes the basis for developing an ethical identity. When the group ideal is shared by its members it also strengthens cohesion and adherence to the group's moral code.

While guilt is object-related, to do with actions harming an "other", shame is self-related and reflects a failure regarding the self. A person can feel guilty for what he does and shame for who he is. These two affects can be jointly experienced as, for example, a man may hurt his brother and feel both guilty for doing so and ashamed that he was unable to control himself. Shame is manifest in a visual perception of the self, reflecting the betrayal of the ideal image of the self; it needs to be hidden from the eyes of others. Guilt is a betrayal of an internalized ideal code of actions that also forms part of the ego ideal. In the case of guilt, however, it is the behavior, not the person, that is condemned.

Shame and the Other

Augustine in his *Confessions* makes the distinction between *facinus* (criminal) and *flagitium* (shame). The criminal is original sin, our propensity to evil. Guilt is tied to the breaking of rules or laws and results from a destructive act. The evaluation of shame, on the other hand, is determined by circumstance. In *De doctrina Christiana*, Augustine writes:

> Because it is shameful (*flagitiose*) to strip the body naked at a banquet among the drunken and licentious, it does not follow that it is shameful (*flagitium*) to be naked in the baths ... We must, therefore, consider carefully what is suitable to times and places and persons, and not rashly charge men with sins (*flagitia*).
>
> (quoted in Ginzburg, p.41)

Augustine makes the point that shame is circumstantial insofar as it occurs when there is a failure in controlling one's behavior in accordance with social expectations or norms. This is not a crime, as Augustine emphasizes, but it can be regarded as an example of human weakness that is involuntary and therefore shameful, if not also demeaning. Shame derives from a humiliation of the self as seen through the eyes of others when a violation of social values is exposed. It is self-referential; it is the evaluation of the self, of the nature and being of the self, rather than actions of the self in relation to others that is at stake. While someone who is guilty of committing a crime may feel regret, they may nevertheless retain a positive view of themselves in other respects. Shame, on the other hand, permeates a sense of one's self, contaminating one's self-image completely, as a flaw reveals a basic problem with the whole. Both guilt and shame are contingent on social precepts with the essential difference that guilt entails self-agency, an action that has been committed knowingly and intentionally by the perpetrator, whereas shame results from a lack of self-agency. It is this lack that marks shame as such a painful experience.

Shame, Attachment and Identity

The fact that shame is determined by social context and relations means that it inevitably plays a central role in an individual's attachment to a group and in the identity this confers. Ginzburg stresses that "shame embodies the relationship between the individual body and the political body" (Ginzburg, p.40). The individual and the group are inextricably linked in the collective sense of honor held within the group that shapes its identity. The individual ego ideal is in accord with the ideal of the group – it is this bond that strengthens the identity of the group. Ginzburg refers to the wider, and more positive, meaning of shame (*aidos*) in ancient Greek as including "honour", "respect", "fear" and "veneration". In the Illiad, Nestor urges his soldiers to fight and says,

> Friends, be men, and set in your heart *(thumos)* shame (*aidos*) for other men, and remember, each of you, your children and wives and property and parents, both those of you whose parents are alive and those whose parents are dead.
>
> (Ginzburg, p.39)

It is not only the honor of the group that must be protected and upheld but the failure to do so and the resulting shame also binds the group together. Ginzburg notes the connection made by the philosopher, Émile Benveniste, between *aidos* and *nemesis*:

> *Aidos* stands for the collective sense of honour and the obligations it implies for the group. But this feeling is strengthened and these obligations are felt most keenly when collective honour is wounded. At that moment the abused "honour" of all becomes the "shame" of each.
>
> (quoted in Ginzburg, p.38)

In linking *aidos* and *nemesis*, Benveniste points to the capacity of shame to bond the group together in its collective downfall. As in the case of the individual, it is the experience of shame that so powerfully affects the way in which a group perceives itself that cannot be absolved or repudiated as in the case of guilt. The narrator of Starritt's novel, *We Germans*, remarks:

> Shame is not like guilt; it's not a matter of reparations. Those people are dead. The ones who were my age, their children and grandchildren were never born. Shame can't be atoned for; it is a debt that cannot be paid.
>
> (Starritt, 2020, Loc. 1019)

Shame becomes an integral part of the group's identity, a stain that cannot be removed and gives rise to a legacy of contamination. As Ginzburg observes, "... the country one belongs to is not, as the usual rhetoric goes, the one you love but the one you are ashamed of. Shame can be a stronger bond than love" (Ginzburg, p.35).

Adam Michnik, the Polish newspaper editor and former dissident, has also argued:

> that a sense of shame can be the basis of belonging to a nation: "He who is ashamed of Polish sins is a Pole." This radical assertion makes

conscience the foundation of identity, and patriotism is hollow without conscience, too. Patriotism often invokes honor; honor requires conscience; and conscience entails the possibility of shame. If the only permissible emotion is pride, then patriotism is merely chauvinism. Love for one's country may be all the stronger for being troubled, and the country may be the stronger for that kind of love.

(Kohn, 12th November 2019)

Benveniste and Michnik both make the important point that it is by virtue of being a member of a group that the individual experiences either glory (honor) or humiliation (shame) as part of his/her identity. This is a markedly different experience to collective guilt in which a group may be accused and take responsibility for the crimes it has committed. The experience of the individual within this group may vary widely depending on how they perceive their degree of culpability. It is certainly not accepted homogeneously by all. This suggests that shame, which is conferred on each member of the group, affects the identity of the whole in a way that collective guilt cannot. As an American, for example, I do not feel guilty for the atrocities committed by the US military during the Vietnam War but, equally, as an American, I do feel shame that I am part of culture that allowed such things to happen.

In the final days of World War Two, the German narrator of Starritt's novel, *We Germans*, reflects:

I also thought: once this war is won, we, like other nations, will have to think about the abhorrent things some of our millions of people perpetrated while it was going on. I wrongly thought that this cruelty was in the individuals, not, fundamentally, in our system of government, in our culture, in us.

A lot has been said about collective guilt. I can't find any holes in the concept – that even if all you did in the war was serve lunches at a quiet rubber factory in the middle of Germany, your meals fed workers whose rubber went into tyres that were fitted to trucks that carried people to their deaths.

No matter how far you were from it, you incurred guilt, in a greater or lesser portion. The only exceptions were those few who refused to work or answer the draft, whom the country is now so grateful to have had. But if you weren't a hero, you colluded by default. Morally, there was no neutral ground, no safe middle of the herd. And I didn't make lunches; I wore a uniform and fought, to the best of my ability.

So I can't fault the concept of our collective guilt, I just don't feel it. The idea that I'm guilty for things I never saw and had no power over doesn't seem to me to meet the standards of natural justice. But what I do feel, ineradicably, is shame.

(Starritt, Loc. 1005–14)

This collective experience of shame, as distinct from guilt, is powerfully depicted by Primo Levi in writing about the opening of the Lager to Russian soldiers, who were the first outsiders to witness what had happened within the camp.

> They did not greet us, nor smile; they seemed oppressed, not only by pity but also by a confused restraint which sealed their mouths, and kept their eyes fastened on the funereal scene. It was the same shame which we knew so well, which submerged us after the selections, and every time we had to witness or undergo an outrage: the shame that the Germans never knew, the shame which the just man experiences when confronted by a crime committed by another, and he feels remorse because of its existence, because of its having been irrevocably introduced into the world of existing things, and because his will has proven nonexistent or feeble and was incapable of putting up a good defence.
>
> (Levi, 1989, p.54)

What is shameful is precisely that man's "will has proven nonexistent" and this is what differentiates the experience from one of guilt.

Our capacity for shame not only binds us together and strengthens our collective identity but, as we can see from Levi's description of the Russian soldiers' reactions, it also opens the way for us to identify with others outside our own group and to recognize the fluidity of our identities and our larger, human identity. Returning to Ginzburg's thoughts about the boundaries of the ego, he notes:

> To speak of every human being having two bodies (the physical and the social, the visible and the invisible) is insufficient. It is more helpful to consider the individual as the point of convergence of multiple sets. We simultaneously belong to a species (*Homo sapiens*), a sex, a linguistic community, a political community, a professional community, and so on and so forth. Ultimately we come across a set, defined by ten finger-prints, which has just one member: ourselves. To define an individual on the basis of his or her fingerprints certainly makes sense in some con-texts. But an individual cannot be identified with his or her unique fea-tures. To achieve a fuller understanding of an individual's deeds and thoughts, present or past, we have to explore the interaction among the sets, specific and generic, to which he or she belongs. The emotion I started from – being ashamed for somebody different from us, for something we are not involved in – is a clue that helps us to rethink our multiple identities, their interaction and their unity, from an unexpected angle.
>
> (Ginzburg, p.44)

Shame, because it marks a lack of agency, provides a mirror to ourselves and to others, a self-awareness that connects us to others that guilt, based on a binary, us-them, paradigm, cannot do. This was the paradox that Adam and Eve came to know.

Shame and Violence

Ginzburg describes the experience of shame as something that "falls upon us", without self-agency. Even if we try to hide our shame from others, we cannot hide it from ourselves; it continues to exist as a painful wound within our self-consciousness. It naturally follows that any attempt to obliterate or expunge shame would inevitably require a powerful act of will, an act that re-establishes a sense of self-agency through the reversal of roles or a process of identification with the aggressor. The experience of shame requires our weakness or failing to be perceived by someone else and it is often inflicted by someone else who has greater power over us, as in any form of abuse. This initial perception is then internalized psychically in the form of exposure to an internal observer who inflicts shame. In an abusive situation, the victim may subsequently try to inflict harm on someone else in order to transpose his shame onto them. Alternatively, the victim may self-abuse in identification with the aggressor, further shaming himself. In this way, the victim-turned-perpetrator attempts to regain a sense of potency and pride, or at the very least, agency.

The forensic psychiatrist, Jim Gilligan, argues that the emotion of shame is the underlying and most significant "cause of all violence, whether towards others or towards the self" (Gilligan, 2000a, p.110). When shame is first evoked, it leads to rage against the impotence inflicted on the self. Our prisons are full of men and women who have histories of humiliation and disrespect; gang warfare is all about keeping face and which gang is more powerful. On a collective level, ongoing political conflicts become intransi-gent against a background of shame with few opportunities of regaining pride.

The psychological weakness of using violence as an antidote to shame is that it comes at a cost; the very act of violence, unless it is intended in self-defense, incurs shame on the perpetrator and this, more than anything else, fuels cycles of violence. The torturer who deliberately sets out to dehumanize his victim must also treat himself as inhuman in order to obliterate the humanness of an "other". When shame is split off and projected onto the "other", this process creates the conditions for a perverse omnipotent structure that has to be maintained as a defense against reality. Experiencing shame may be so overwhelming that it is perceived as life threatening.

Within this perverse system, shame is defended against through further violence and becomes self-perpetuating. Shameful feelings are normalized and transformed into a perverse ideal. A clear example of this can be seen in an excerpt from a film episode about the Chernobyl nuclear power disaster that left much of the local population of humans and animals fatally contaminated. A young man volunteers to clear different areas of human and animal life as a means of containing contaminants. An older, more experienced volunteer spurs his younger colleague to shoot a dog in a farmyard in accord with party orders. The younger man struggles to do so and eventually succeeds. It is clear that he does not feel guilty, after all he was following orders, so much as ashamed of killing a helpless animal in cold blood. The older man tries to comfort him and says,

> Look … this happens to everyone their first time. Normally, when you kill a man, but for you, a dog. So what? There's no shame in it … My first time, Afghanistan. We were moving toward a house then suddenly a man was there and I shot him in the stomach. Yeah, that's a real war story. There are never any good stories, like in the movies. They're shit. A man was there – boom, stomach. I was so scared I didn't pull the trigger again for the rest of the day. I thought, "Well, that's it, Bacho. You put a bullet in someone. You're not you anymore. You'll never be you again." But then you wake up the next morning and you're still you. And you realise … that was you all along. You just didn't know.
> (Chernobyl, Season 1, Ep. 4: 'The Happiness of All Mankind')

A patient of mine, a Vietnam veteran, described a similar experience after he had shot in cold blood a man whom he thought was with the Viet Cong.

> He suddenly ran towards me out of the bush. He wasn't carrying any weapon, or at least I couldn't see anything, and looked terrified. I remember thinking, either I shoot him or I risk being killed – but it wasn't clear. I was terrified, terrified of shooting him and terrified of being shot. I decided to shoot and he fell down in front of me, dying. It was the first time. I was in shock and couldn't believe I had killed a man, I couldn't believe it was me, the same me who believed I was good. I felt contaminated, like a stain had seeped through my whole being and would never go away, never fade. Strangely, I did not feel guilty – I told myself, at least, that I was defending myself, I was a soldier at the front and I had acted under orders – but I felt dirtied and ashamed. I had lost my innocence and I knew I would do this again and that the shame would always be there no matter what. It was not something I could ever feel proud about – like some of the guys who would boast about how many "Charlies" they had downed. But it also became normal – to kill – and each time I knew I had killed someone, I felt a sense of satisfaction. It was a satisfaction in knowing I had done my job well but at another level it also confirmed that the "gooks" weren't the same as us, they weren't really human like us and this meant I had nothing to be ashamed of.

At this point my patient broke down in tears and explained that he had never admitted these things to anyone.

My patient's description of how he managed his shame is a striking account of how atrocities are normalized when violence becomes a means of obliterating guilt. However, the leftover cognitive dissonance of believing oneself to be good and doing something bad is unbearable. The shame arising from inflicting violence can only be mitigated by allegiance to fellow perpetrators. Martens points out:

> ... after individuals have killed a number of times, they cross a "threshold" of killing, or a "point of no return." At this point it is no longer psychologically acceptable or viable for individuals to view their killing as shameful, and so they engage in further killing to convince themselves and others that the killing was warranted and permissible in the first place.
>
> (Martens et al., 2010, p.268, quoted in Mitton, 2015, p.163)

The manipulation of shame within violent contexts is a common strategy in maintaining a perpetrator culture and perverse systems of power. David Keen comments:

> For example, recruitment of fighters may rest on exploiting and exacerbating shame, while legitimizing abusive war systems may depend on *distributing* shame in particular ways. A striking feature of shame and guilt is that perpetrators frequently feel remarkably little of either (seeing their own violence as justified or even righteous), while the victims of violence – including sexual violence – often feel great shame and guilt, even though they have done nothing wrong.
>
> (Keen, 2012, p.197)

The victim becomes the scapegoat for the perpetrator's shame and guilt. Cleansing of shame and guilt can then only be managed by committing further violence. This is equally the case with victims who may also resort to violence as a means of expelling shame; in this way the cycle of violence and revenge escalates.[4]

Mitton's research on atrocities committed in the Sierra Leone civil war similarly revealed that amongst the perpetrators,

> guilt was markedly absent ... As Gilligan has observed: "no one feels as innocent as the criminals; their lack of guilt feelings, even over the most atrocious of crimes, is one of their most prominent characteristics" (Gilligan, 2001, p.113). Shame, however, is strongly related to self-worth, rather than innocence ... "a deep lack of self-worth based on the dread of being unmasked as worthless" (Whittington, 2007, p.312).
>
> (Mitton, p.116)

While guilt can be eliminated through various justifications, principally through the group's licensing of violence, shame is a different matter because it is connected to self-worth. Shame binds the group together in a way that guilt cannot.[5] Shaming rituals, for example the humiliations that are an integral part of many initiation rites, create powerful bonds to the group out of the need to restore self-esteem and counteract being helpless. Through shaming, the group establishes its power over the individual and can then offer protection and a coherent identity. Gilligan notes that perpetrators of violence will "sacrifice anything to prevent the death and disintegration of their individual or group identity" (Gilligan, p.97). The added and underlying element of shame that is shared within the group reinforces allegiance to the group as it offers the promise of self-agency and restoration of power.

Just as shame can be used to reinforce group identity, it can also be used to fuel hatred of what is seen to be an established social order. Atrocities are often regarded as a symptom of the breakdown of social order rather than as an attack on a social order that has become the target of groups that need to identify an "other" to wreak revenge and shame upon. The trauma of being shamed makes the individual (or group) especially defensive and paradoxically more vulnerable to manipulation when it comes to retaliatory violence. René Girard makes the important point that "when unappeased, violence seeks and always finds a surrogate victim. The creature that excited its fury is abruptly replaced by another, chosen only because it is vulnerable and close at hand" (quoted in Mitton, p.118). Whittington argues further that this attempt to eliminate humiliation by reversing the roles of victim and aggressor can only provide temporary relief to the perpetrator as the original shaming episode is never addressed directly but continues to be repressed and enacted in reverse. The result is the perpetrator becomes caught in an addictive cycle of violence. As Whittington explains, "Revenge becomes an end in itself, a need for discharge, upon whom it does not matter" (quoted in Mitton, p.118). These cycles of shame are especially evident in conflicts that continue across generations, feuds that cannot be resolved as they are being constantly renewed and relived over time.

Cultures of Shame and Cultures of Guilt

The social anthropologist, Ruth Benedict, was amongst the first to coin the terms, "guilt culture" and "shame culture", claiming that there is a clear distinction between the two. In June 1944, the month when the Battle of Normandy was launched in World War Two and American forces landed in Saipan, Benedict was employed by the US government to produce a cultural analysis of Japan to understand how the Japanese, as enemies of the US and its Allies, would behave in war. Questions such as whether the Japanese would fight to the end, how to deal with and understand the role of the emperor, and what problems might be encountered by Allied occupation after the war were key to US military decision making. Benedict had never been to Japan and conducted much of her research through a variety of sources including literature, film, foreigners writing about Japan, and from contact with Japanese people living in the US at the time. Benedict's "armchair" analysis is remarkable in its depth and freedom from stereotypical foreign views of the Japanese. She has been latterly criticized for her assumption that it is possible to describe a "national character" and yet her emphasis on the importance of national identity and what this means in terms of national behavior remains highly relevant today. Most importantly, her study highlights the significant role that a nation's ideals play in shaping the history and identity of its citizens.

Benedict defined a guilt culture as a "society that inculcates absolute standards of morality and relies on man's developing a conscience." A shame culture, in contrast, is evident when "people are chagrined about acts which we expect people to feel guilty about", adding that this

> chagrin cannot be relieved, as guilt can be, by confession and atonement ... (A) man does not experience relief when he makes his fault public even to a confessor. So long as his bad behaviour does not 'get out into the world' he need not be troubled and confession appears to him merely a way of courting trouble.
>
> (quoted in Buruma, 1994, p.116)

These distinctions reveal a number of problems and prejudices, the most obvious one being her phrase "developing a conscience" that suggests that guilt is a more advanced moral emotion than shame, which is only activated if the bad behavior is observed by someone else; otherwise shame can remain dormant with no effect on the person concerned. Benedict's point that guilt can be atoned for and absolved whereas "chagrin cannot be relieved" in this manner is at the nub of the matter. Guilt can be relieved because it is an act; shame taints the person irrevocably because it is to do with self-worth.

In the examples I have given, the distinction Benedict makes between shame and guilt now appears to be simplistic, if not moralistic. As research in infant development demonstrates, shame and guilt can coexist, but they are of a different order. Benedict's study does, however, raise questions about the kinds of ideals that groups aspire to and how these become manifest in culture. There are some interesting parallels – and differences – in comparing Japan's Emperor Hirohito to Hitler. In his book, *Wages of Guilt*, Buruma describes the lethal consequences of the emperor-worship culture in Japan, a culture that seemed to be leading to national suicide at the end of the war. Buruma writes:

> A veteran of the war in China said in a television interview that he was able to kill Chinese without qualms only because he didn't regard them as human. There was even religious merit in the killing, for it was part of a

"holy war." Captain Francis P. Scott, the chaplain at Sugamo prison, questioned Japanese camp commandants about their reasons for mistreating POWs. This is how he summed up their answers: "They had a belief that any enemy of the emperor could not be right, so the more brutally they treated their prisoners, the more loyal to their emperor they were being."

(Buruma, p.173)

What the war veteran describes, and how the Japanese camp commandants justified their cruelty towards POWs, bears a striking resemblance to accounts made by Hitler's followers. In both cultures, the leader had been internalized as an omnipotent figure who could do no wrong and who demanded unquestioning loyalty in return for unconditional love. The psychology was similar. Buruma comments:

> The Mitscherlichs described Hitler as an object on which Germans depended, to which they transferred responsibility, and he was thus an internal object. As such, he represented and revived the ideas of omnipotence that we all cherish about ourselves from infancy. The same was true of the Japanese imperial institution, no matter who sat on the throne, a ruthless war criminal or a gentle marine biologist.

(Buruma, p.173)

While the histories of both countries differ, a similar dynamic was constellated and exacerbated under existential threat. Hitler was able to take advantage of Germany's past humiliations by promising a return to omnipotence under his leadership. It was past shame that fueled a new group supremacy. Japan, on the other hand, had a tradition of emperor worship that bestowed a sense of supremacy over the population as compared with foreigners or outsiders. The belief of supremacy strengthens the ties within the group along with its identity and stresses the ideal of supporting the emperor at all costs. Pride and honor – what the ancient Greeks referred to as *Aidos* – are especially valued. Any weakness that is revealed by a member of the group or by the group itself is experienced as a narcissistic failing that brings shame on everyone. Because the godlike emperor can do no wrong, this means that the group can do no wrong – its actions can cause no harm because it is always in the right, like Buruma's reference to a "holy war". Shame, however, is the pre-eminent emotion as it comes from a loss of face. It was also shame, rather than guilt, that we see behind the suicides at the end of Hitler's Reich. While, within our Judeo-Christian tradition, we may feel that each country *should* feel guilt because of the war crimes they committed, is this in fact our way of distancing ourselves even further from our own sense of shame?[6] In pointing the finger of guilt at perpetrators as a group – and in our assumption that guilt indicates a more mature response to acts of violence – are we hoping that we can restore our ideal of social and moral order without having to acknowledge that shame is the problem that lives on and cannot be atoned for?

Conclusion

In his study of shame, the philosopher, Bernard Williams, states, "We can feel both guilt and shame towards the same action" (Williams, 1993, p.92). He makes the distinction that guilt derives from an action that has to do with "what has happened to others", specifically, harming others, and shame derives from the effect of these actions on "what I am" (Ibid.). This is the dual experience of the perpetrator I have referred to. Williams includes in the category of guilt involuntary actions or those actions that we have not voluntarily taken but nevertheless implicate us morally, often in the form of a failure to act or intervene that makes us complicit in someone else's harm. Williams argues, however, that

> The conception of modern morality … insist at once on the primacy of guilt, its significance in turning us towards victims, and its rational restriction to the voluntary … In fact, if we want to understand why it might be important for us to distinguish the harms we do voluntarily from those that we do involuntarily, we shall hope to succeed only if we ask what kinds of failing or inadequacy are the source of the harms, and what those failings mean in the context of our own and other people's lives. This is the territory of shame; it is only by moving into it that we may gain some insight into one of the main preoccupations of the morality that centres itself on guilt.
>
> (Ibid., p.94)

Williams is making the important point that while guilt is associated with breaking collective social rules, shame reflects the basis, often unconscious, of our personal internal morality. While the observer of a shameful act or a condition of shame may be someone else or a group that one belongs to, the observer is also present within the individual psyche when the ego fails to conform to the ego ideal, as in the expression, "I have let myself down". Williams continues to argue that guilt

> leaves out a lot even of one's ethical consciousness. It can direct one towards those who have been wronged or damaged, and demand reparation in the name, simply, of what has happened to them. But it cannot by itself help one to understand one's relations to those happenings, or to rebuild the self that has done these things and the world in which that self has to live. Only shame can do that, because it embodies conceptions of what one is and of how one is related to others.
>
> (Ibid., p.94)

Returning to the idea of original sin in Christianity, God can absolve a person, through the ritual of Baptism, of the original sin committed by Adam and Eve of disobeying Him but He cannot remove the human condition of shame. The theology is clear that sin is always a personal act and cannot be inherited or passed on to others, but shame is shared by all as our awareness of our own susceptibility to and capacity for corruption. Insofar as shame is a loss of self-agency it also points to a lapse of will as we are taken over by emotional forces that override our moral consciousness. Primo Levi eloquently describes this condition:

> And there is another, vaster shame, the shame of the world ... It was not possible for us, nor did we want, to become islands; the just among us, nei- ther more nor less numerous than in any other human group, felt remorse, shame and pain for the misdeeds that others and not they had com- mitted, and in which they felt involved, because they sensed that what had happened around them in their presence, and in them, was irrevoc- able. It would never again be able to be cleansed; it would prove that man, the human species – we, in short – were potentially able to construct an infinite enormity of pain ...
>
> (Levi, "Shame", pp.65–6)

Levi describes the shame we experience, as humans, when we are faced with the misdeeds of others, shame from our awareness that we too are guilty of such destructiveness. Arendt goes a step further and is concerned with what this means in terms of our responsibility towards one another as human beings. She is clear that "men must assume responsibility for all crimes com- mitted by men and that all nations share the onus of evil committed by all others" (Arendt, 1994, p.131). Arendt is not saying that men should feel guilty for all crimes committed by men but that they must assume responsi- bility for what has happened. Arendt would consider this an act of self-agency which, as such, is always a political function. This brings us into the realm of our political and social responsibilities going forward into the future; it does not extend to taking on the guilt of others. Arendt goes on to argue that "Shame at being a human being is the purely individual and still non-political expression of this insight" (Ibid.). Arendt's understanding of shame is that it is a personal experience, it is bound directly to one's self-image and in this respect it is not an abstract or intellectual acknowledgement. Shame is a "non-political expression" because it does not lead to action, it remains internal, as an acknowledgement of a failing, of a lack of will. Only the acknowledgement of responsibility, as a derivation of shame, can be expressed politically.

This brings us full circle to Williams's point that understanding our shame will enable us to "better understand our guilt." Williams writes, "The struc- tures of shame contain the possibility of controlling and learning from guilt, because they give a conception of one's ethical identity, in relation to which guilt can make sense. Shame can understand guilt, but guilt cannot understand itself" (Williams, p.93). Through our experience of shame, we gain an awareness of our own moral position not only towards others but within ourselves.

Notes

1 Victims of the nuclear bomb attacks in Hiroshima and Nagasaki were referred to as "Hibakusha" and, along with their children, discriminated against socially and economically. Hibakusha were shunned as marriage prospects and had difficulty in obtaining employment and medical care.
2 In Latin, the word for apple, *malum*, also means evil.
3 A more primitive form of shame, described by Carvalho as "ontological shame", may be experienced in infancy when there is a premature and severe disjunction between the infant's signaled need/desire and the environmental response, creating an acute sense of helplessness and exposure or "nakedness". The infant does not have a conscious sense of agency at this early stage but the failure of response is experienced and remembered emotionally as a narcissistic wound that results in a deep sense of unworthiness, later expressed as shame relating to one's being. This is distinct from shame accrued later in development that derives from social perceptions of the self in which there is a failure in self-agency that exposes the ego's vulnerability before others' eyes. (Personal communication from Richard Carvalho)
4 This dynamic of violence fueled by mounting guilt and shame has been widely recognized in descriptions of the KL system under the German Third Reich by Primo Levi and others. (See also, Sofsky, W. (1993). *The Order of Terror: The Concentration Camp*. Princeton: Princeton University Press.)
5 Shame also binds perpetrators to their victims in their role as carriers for their own shame and humiliation.
6 It is possible that due to Germany's Judeo-Christian tradition it was more amenable to acknowledging guilt than seemed to be the case in Japan. Beneath the surface, shame has nevertheless played an important part in both cultures.

References

Arendt, H. (1994). *Essays in Understanding: 1930–1954*. New York: Schocken Books.
Bachmann, I. (2018). *War Diary*. London: Seagull Books.
Benedict, R. (2005). *The Chrysanthemum and the Sword*. New York: A Mariner Book, Houghton Mifflin Company.
Bible, King James' version.
Buruma, I. (1994). *The Wages of Guilt: Memories of War in Germany and Japan*. London: Atlantic Books.
Gilligan, J. (2000a). *Violence: Reflections on our Deadliest Epidemic*. London: Jessica Kingsley Publishers.
Ginzburg, C. (Nov/Dec 2019). "The Bond of Shame." *New Left Review*, 120, pp.35–44.
Keen, D. (2012). *Useful Enemies: When Waging Wars is More Important than Winning Them*. London: Yale University Press.

Kohn, M. (12 November 2019). "From Lublin to London, Europe's Contested Ideas of National Identity." *New York Review of Books Daily.*

Levi, P. (1989). *The Drowned and the Saved.* London: Abacus.

Mazin, C. (2019). *Chernobyl*, Season 1, Ep.4: The Happiness of All Mankind

Mitton, K. (2015). *Rebels in a Rotten State: Understanding Atrocity in Sierra Leone.* London: Hurst & Company.

Starritt, A. (2020). *We Germans.* London: J M Originals.

Velleman, J.D. (2001). "The Genesis of Shame." *Philosophy & Public Affairs*, 30(1).

Williams, B. (1993). *Shame and Necessity.* Berkeley: University of California Press.

Chapter 5

Saving Face
Memory, Identity and Blame

> Every time I talk about the past, it's a different story. It's not about what really happened, it's about what story I can live with in the present.
>
> (Simon, writer)

Memory and History

We make sense of our lives, we create and recreate our identity, through our construction of the past, a narrative that explains how our present emotional and physical state derives from a sequence of events that, put together, form a causal chain. We naturally structure our perception of our lives in terms of beginnings, middles and ends – a storyline that reinforces the idea that we have a continuous and consistent experience of self that, inevitably shaped by the joys and traumas in our lives, constitutes what we call our identity. We also know that the narrative we construct is not altogether factual either, because we cannot know the facts due to the limits and distortions of memory or because we are selective about the facts we recall, siphoning off the ones that do not fit into our narrative.

One of the earliest and most famous life stories is that of Odysseus, starting with his departure from his homeland, Ithaca, to fight in the Trojan War. The adventures and struggles Odysseus encounters are often described as illustrating a process of individuation in which Odysseus discovers aspects of himself that transform him from serving as a tool of the gods to becoming a man able to exercise his own agency. While this is the archetypal narrative structure of the hero's tale, it is also an ideal model that we strive for in describing our lives. The goal of psychoanalytic work is bound to this ideal – to understand one's limitations and potential and in doing so to alter one's perception of oneself from helpless victim to having the agency to direct one's life.[1] Memory, whether it is individual or collective, is the primary means by which we establish who we are, what happened to us, how we imagine our future and what we need to survive, both materially and ontologically. It is our perception of our past and how we understand this that shapes our present and our future.

DOI: 10.4324/9781003379980-6

The French historian, Pierre Nora, states, "The quest for memory is the search for one's history" (Nora, 1989, p.13). In this deceptively simple statement, Nora opens different levels of meaning about history and memory and the various questions that come out of this. We experience memory as not only personal but fluid, unreliable, and selective; different people witnessing or involved in the same event are likely to remember it differently. Whether it is individual or collective memory, remembering is to do with putting together bits of the past into a pattern that is not static or fixed but shifts as our brains adapt and absorb our perceptions in the present. History, on the other hand, connotes a shared understanding of an event, albeit also subject to revision over time. In marking the difference between memory and history, Gregorio Kohon, a psychoanalyst, writes, "While memory of the past ties us to the present, taking root in personal spaces, gestures, images and objects, history is a representation of the past that 'belongs to everyone and to no one'" (Kohon, 2021, p.5). Because history is a shared narrative, it becomes a witness to memory, validating (and forming) our perceptions of what has happened. In this respect, the process of psychoanalysis could be described as transforming memory into history as the role of the analyst is to provide a witness to the remembered events as they emerge in analysis and to the internal events experienced within the psychic reality of the patient. Without a witness, memory not only remains in the realm of the personal but, even more significantly, it lies within the uncertain space between fantasy and truth. Once witnessed, personal memory becomes personal history; this history can then be incorporated within the patient's self-narrative. The process of creating a narrative that is shared or witnessed provides the essential foundation for creating a sense of self-agency; I am the one who tells my story, not others. As master of the past, the storyteller is given mastery over the present and the future.

The shared memories that bind us together in creating a common history are, however, not to be confused with fact or truth. History, as we are aware, inevitably represents the interests and experiences of the individual or group as they see it. It is not the only story but it is normally the selected story that best serves the interests of the group.[2] As with the construction of a life narrative, history is founded largely on causal, linear principles that shape and reinforce individual and collective identity. For example, we are used to analyzing the causes of war in terms of deliberate actions or reactions determined by events, as consciously driven. The reality, as we often discover, is that war may be caused by chance events and failures of communication that have had disastrous consequences. A series of blunders does not make for a good story and certainly does not reinforce our wish to believe that we are able, at least to some degree, to determine our fate. When things go wrong, when mistakes occur, when leadership fails, group identity is protected by placing blame on the "other", thereby preserving its sense of purity and being in the right.

Professor Vamik Volkan, a psychoanalyst who founded the study of political psychology, coined the term "chosen trauma" to connote a mental representation of a massive trauma shared by a large group over generations to consolidate group identity and to establish the group's historical narrative. Alongside the "chosen trauma" is also the "chosen glory" that celebrates the strength of the group and bolsters self-esteem. When the group's existence is threatened, its chosen trauma is reactivated as a warning of danger and to instill aggression against the "other", the enemy. Although the "chosen trauma" serves to strengthen group identity in times of crisis, it may have destructive consequences if it is used to reframe and distort history for political purposes. What is memorialized and what is vilified in a country's history, especially in relation to war, civil and otherwise, shapes its identity and future relations with others, particularly in establishing which groups are considered "good" and which "bad". The debate in the US about Civil War memorials is a case in point, as is the heated debate in the UK that has led to the deposition of the Cecil Rhodes statue at Oxford University amongst others.

Saving Face and Maintaining Power

The narrative we establish for ourselves, whether individually or collectively, is not only created to make sense of who we are in relation to others and to assert our moral position in the world, it also saves face. We portray ourselves as either victims, heroes, repentant sinners, or helpless bystanders. As individuals we naturally want to place ourselves in these roles when we remember the past because, apart from our own self-esteem and internal moral conscience, we want to demonstrate our "goodness" to reaffirm our value as a member of our group, as belonging to society. Individual histories are inevitably subjective and self-serving. The self-image of the group, however, has greater significance as it is what holds the group together and ensures its moral/social survival. It is especially important for group identity then to select what events to memorialize from its past and how to depict these events – either as "chosen traumas" or as "chosen glories".

W.G. Sebald, in writing about the silence following the German civilian experience of war, observes: "When we turn to take a retrospective view we are always looking and looking away at the same time" (Sebald, 2003). This statement highlights what we are doing when we look at the past, as if there is a "real" past to be seen, not that the process of looking itself is necessarily through some form of lens that is deeply connected to how we see ourselves or want to be seen. This does not mean that the way the past is depicted or remembered is intentionally or consciously manipulated. What we fail to see from the past may not be due to denial or censorship but may be determined by other factors, such as the conditions in which an event takes place. Alexander Starritt describes the political happenstance of memory in writing about the German atrocities in Russia:

In the first year in the East, we Germans starved two and a half million Russian prisoners to death, intentionally. I have seen a man starve to death, I have starved, and it isn't painless, it's not some dull lethargy. It's frantic. Just that, that alone, out of all that was done, was a crime that requires monuments and speeches and days of mourning, but because it was perpetrated in the East, it is hardly remembered.

(Starritt, 2020, Loc. 966–71)

Whatever reason is ascribed to the fact that certain events are excised from our collective memory, the "chosen" memory that achieves precedence at different points in time invariably reflects the self-image the group wishes to inculcate within its members and to the world at large. The object of saving face, which is evident in every political exchange and interpretation of events, requires the manipulation of the "truth" to appear to accord to mutually recognized moral beliefs. No group wants to accept blame for harming others, but when this is unavoidable the group will attempt to restore its moral rectitude by different means, for example, either in a defensive way – there was no other viable choice or the group is being victimized – or by acknowledging the harm done and promising reparation. Saving face is paramount for the group to retain its power, its alliances, and to be seen to be acting within a universally accepted moral code.

What is forgotten is as significant as what is remembered. It is abundantly clear that monuments and memorials are created not only to signify what is important in the life of the group, as either trauma or glory, but to present a purified, moral face to the public, whether it is as innocent victims or as triumphant victors who have fought against injustice. Whatever is memorialized presents a kind of "selfie" to the world of how the group in power sees itself and its relations to others. Monuments celebrate the group in power and in doing so can also be used to perpetuate its power. One notable example is the proliferation of monuments that have been erected in Rwanda following the genocide. In this period Rwanda's president, Paul Kagame, has not only extended his term of office but has used commemoration of the genocide to strengthen his position further, especially with regard to cleansing the government of its enemies.

The Kigali Genocide Memorial, along with six other major centers in Rwanda, was established to commemorate the victims of the 1994 genocide, some 250,000 of whom are buried in mass graves beneath its foundation. The message from the Rwandan Patriotic Front, in power for more than two decades, echoes the mantra, "Never Again", at the gates of Auschwitz. The Memorial signifies the tragedy of the genocide and Rwanda's recovery through, as Rwanda expert Michela Wrong describes it, "a benign technocrat who rebuilt a traumatized state and miraculously delivered peace, stability, and economic growth rates routinely exceeding 5 percent each year" (Wrong, 2016).

However, since these memorial sites were created, new museums have appeared that are delivering a more subtle and troubling authoritarian message. These museums, located in the former homes and headquarters of the rich, illustrate in gruesome detail what happens to those dissidents who threaten to overpower the government. One example of a popular museum of this sort is the villa of former President Juvénal Habyarimana in Kigali, opened as the Presidential Museum in 2009. Wrong writes:

> Habyarimana, an army chief of staff who led a presidential coup in 1973, lived in paranoid anticipation that his own turn would come: His palace is a mini-fortress equipped with motion sensors on its stairs and a fake wall in a TV room that opens to reveal a concealed rifle rack and secret staircase—an escape route for his family. Habyarimana famously perished alongside his Burundian counterpart when a jet they were traveling in was shot down in April 1994, the event that triggered the genocide. The plane fell right next to the presidential villa, which lies in an elegant Kigali suburb underneath the main flight path into the capital's airport. A British TV crew that visited the site soon after the double assassination spotted what looked like human brains spattered on Habyarimana's Mercedes-Benz. Today, the plane's twisted, rusting debris still sits where it crashed, just outside the villa's garden walls. Museum visitors can wander around it as they please. So can the Rwandan couples who choose the villa as a venue for their wedding receptions, often held in a marquee on the lawn.
>
> (Wrong, 2016)[3]

Although Kagame denies that the RPF was behind Habyarimana's assassination, a Human Rights Watch report from 2014 states that the Rwandan government "does not tolerate opposition, challenge, or criticism" and uses "arbitrary arrests, detentions, prosecutions, killings, torture, enforced disappearances, threats, harassment, and intimidation against government opponents and critics" (quoted in Wrong, 2016).[4]

Kagame, like most modern-day leaders, supports the imperative, as he expresses it, "We must know where we come from to know where we are going." This statement is, however, fraught with interpretive complexity. "Where we come from" does not have the same meaning for everyone, especially if we, for example, look at the differences in Rwanda alone between the history of the Hutus, the Tutsis and the region as a whole. Depending on how "where we come from" is understood, it will indeed affect the country's idea of "where we are going", or perhaps more specifically, "where it *should* be going." The seemingly contradictory message given by these different memorial sites is essentially, "the way to overcome mass violence and atrocities and to achieve peace is by supporting the authoritarian regime in power."

With the right emphasis or "spin", culpability can be transformed and the power of the state reinforced. Svetlana Alexievich describes this process in the aftermath of the Chernobyl nuclear disaster. Referring to the firemen who courageously battled the explosion without being aware of the lethal effects of radiation exposure, she writes:

> Today, they are dying; but what if they had not done what they did? I consider them the heroes, not the casualties of a war which supposedly never happened. They call it "an accident", "a disaster", but it was a war. Our Chernobyl monuments resemble war memorials.
>
> (Alexievich, 2016, pp.176–7)

The incompetence and deceit of the Soviet government was masked as "an accident", "a disaster"; memorials did not mark the lies the government had disseminated about the nuclear power plant, they marked the bravery of those who sacrificed their lives as a result of these lies.[5] By glorifying the firefighters (government employees who were given no choice in this mission), the Kremlin was able eventually to celebrate its own conquest over an accident that it had no power to prevent. We see a similar sleight of hand in the last few years in the Polish government's position in relation to Poland's involvement in the Holocaust. On 1st February 2018, Poland's Senate ratified a bill that outlaws blaming Poland for any crimes committed during the Holocaust. This is one of the most overt examples of any country legislating history and its interpretation in order to appear blameless. It is a crude example of blame being located in "the other", while exonerating the Polish who either had nothing to do with such crimes or were helpless to intervene.

Shifting Blame from Perpetrators to Victims

In attempting to deny involvement in atrocities, groups may also defend themselves by adopting the narrative that they were the real victims, either of an invading force or of prior historical conflicts: they shift the blame to someone else. When the aggressors are attacked, they become the wounded innocent and guilt is projected on to the "other". The "chosen trauma" signifies the group as victim, not as aggressor, and absolves the group of wrongdoing. This process is apparent across cultures and time. In his famous address to the Reichstag on 1st September 1933, declaring the start of World War Two, Hitler accuses the Poles of attacking German territory. He goes a step further to declare that as the enemy "departs from the rules of human warfare", so will Germany in self-defense. Wrongdoing and the blame that accompanies this are projected on to the "other" to maintain the purity of the group.

Shifting blame also comes in other guises. The American withdrawal of military troops from Afghanistan has marked global acknowledgement that US peace-building efforts to secure democratic structures of government in the country over a twenty-year period (the longest US war in history) have failed. While criticisms of US interventionism abound, now that defeat is undisputed, one of the strongest arguments put forward in defense of the US is that it was in fact the Afghans who were not "ready" for democracy. Despite the intensive efforts of the US military and the $143 billion spent on "nation-building", it was the Afghans who failed to accept democracy. As Fintan O'Toole notes, failure is attributed to the Afghans who are "too backward, too poor, too inextricably entangled in medieval tribalism and obscurantist religion" (O'Toole, 2021). These accusations are in a similar vein to blaming an abused and deprived child for not doing well at school; they mask the underlying problem that rather than bringing peace to the region, many critics claim that US intervention only brought further violence.[6] These failings can be understood as common failings in any war, especially when factional conflicts are exacerbated by external forces within a region. However, O'Toole points to the deepest flaw of intervention as lying in the lack of democratic process behind the decision to invade Afghanistan. O'Toole writes:

> From the very beginning, the problem with the US involvement in Afghanistan lay essentially in the deficits in American democracy. A well-functioning republic makes decisions—especially those as serious as starting a war—by an open process of rational deliberation. It asks the obvious questions: What are we doing? Why are we doing it? What is the human and financial cost? What are the benefits? How and when does it end? The original sin of the Afghan war—one that would never be expiated—was the failure of American political institutions to meet these most basic standards of scrutiny.
>
> (O'Toole, 2021)

O'Toole does not account for the shift in perception of the war; it was initially provoked by 9/11 as a defense against further terrorist attacks and only subsequently became a war about nation-building. John Bolton, military advisor to President Bush, is clear in his view that this shift in the way that the Afghan war has been justified has caused problems. Bolton states:

> … We have lost sight of the fact that the main reason for being in Afghanistan was forward defense of the US and its allies to make sure the Taliban didn't resume control and once again offer sanctuary to Al-Qaeda or similar terrorist groups. In my mind it was never a mission to nation-build in Afghanistan and to bring democracy to centralize the government or anything like that, although I think that's what it became and we became part of an Afghan civil war. But that was never our strategic mission and I think loss of that and an unwillingness of America's leadership to explain what the real strategic reason was left people with a feeling that this was a long and futile struggle that we've now abandoned.
>
> (Interview with Jon Snow, Channel 4 News, 31st August 2021)

It is common for narratives to change as we adapt them to our changing realpolitik. These excerpts and comments about the Afghan war illustrate how the rationale shifted over time to accord with the political face-saving of the US and how blame has also shifted from the terrorist organizations to the Afghans themselves to mask the confusion Bolton points out in our understanding of the US mission in Afghanistan. The recent botched American withdrawal from Afghanistan that failed to protect the civilian population and ex-patriots residing there has only served to bring further embarrassment and shame to the US. Biden, a long-term opponent of US involvement, nevertheless failed to apologize for the way in which US withdrawal was handled. Rather than admitting its mistakes, the popular narrative of US involvement in Afghanistan has tended to morph into self-righteousness.

Another form of shifting blame is described by Jelena Subotić as "memory appropriation". Subotić, a political scientist, illustrates this process in detail in the case of Holocaust remembrance practices in Serbia, Croatia, Lithuania and other Eastern European states. She explains,

> ... the memory of the Holocaust is used to memorialize a different kind of suffering, such as suffering under communism, or suffering from ethnic violence perpetrated by other groups. It is Holocaust remembrance turned inward, away from the actual victims of the Holocaust or the Holocaust itself, what Ewa Plonowska Ziaret calls the "narcissistic identification with Jewish suffering."
>
> (Subotić, 2019, p.9)

What Ziaret describes as "narcissistic identification" is not, however, simply identification, it is also used to establish superiority; it is a contest of who has suffered most. It is not in the vein of, "We too have suffered", it is more, "You think you have suffered! What about us!" The hierarchy of suffering is trumped in order to establish which is the most abused group of victims and therefore has the greatest claim to recognition and, in some cases, reparation.[7]

One interpretation of this form of shifting blame by the perpetrator group identifying as the victim is that this is a means of avoiding or denying guilt. However, there is scant evidence that this is the case. Instead, perpetrator groups tend to see themselves as victims when they feel that the acts condoned, if not extolled, in their world have been attacked and their sacrifices debased. This was certainly expressed by many Germans post-Hitler. In writing about atrocities committed in the war in Sierra Leone, the political scientist, Kieran Mitton, comments:

> Perversely, the moral outrage of victims of violence may in itself have provoked moral outrage from their tormentors. In this sense, it was not that victims stirred up dormant or deeply-buried feelings of guilt or shame in perpetrators, but that perpetrators felt angry that actions that

were morally justified and celebrated within the rebel world were being condemned. Combined with anger over perceived civilian betrayal, this may account for the discomforting "genuine sense of outrage and self-righteousness" that Keen observed among many young Sierra Leonean fighters (Keen, 2012a, p. 204).

(quoted in Mitton, 2015, pp.159–60)

In this case, we can say that the perpetrator group's outrage is due to the humiliation of losing face or being shamed in front of the world – and it is in front of a world that does not recognize its "rightful" position.

When groups and their leaders have been accused of serious crimes, affecting the honor and face of the group, it is of vital importance to justify these crimes to remain powerful and "righteous" in the eyes of the members of the group.[8] Leaders who openly acknowledge responsibility – and blame – for their misdeeds and/or those of the group in the present are rare. On the other hand, accepting blame for past crimes may be advantageous in many respects, particularly in the far-off past when the crimes had nothing to do with those alive in the present and when leaders can be seen to attempt to make atonement or reparation and to save face in moral opinion. Accepting blame for harm done in the present is much rarer. This is apparent, for example, in responses to the Black Lives Matter movement in which historic racism has received more public attention than perhaps ever before while racism in the present continues to be denied or adequately addressed.

We can see how adept groups are at shaping their history to bolster their identity and public face and how resistant groups are to accepting blame, much less guilt. Echoing the philosopher George Santayana's dictum, powerful leaders across the world appear to share the belief that it is essential to be aware of history in order not to repeat the mistakes of the past.[9] This is certainly true in the case of individuals – we grow and develop emotionally and intellectually partly through learning from our mistakes. But is this the case with groups?

Not Learning from History

We tend to apply similar moral judgements and expectations to groups as we do to each other as individuals. In our observations of what we see as evidence of collective guilt, and in our efforts to encourage collective atonement and forgiveness, we are not only apportioning blame and innocence and establishing a specific narrative to a set of events, we are also expecting large groups to behave in the same way as an individual might; distinctions between the two collapse. In addition to this, our Judeo-Christian morality, in terms of how we *should* feel and act under certain circumstances, further informs our expectations of group behavior.[10]

The psychoanalytic process as it applies to individuals typically entails stages of initial blame and guilt, validation and witnessing by the analyst, leading to mourning and responsibility, and concluding with acceptance and self-agency. For example, in the case of parental abuse, the childhood trauma is identified and located as deriving from the parents, creating a significant shift from the child's view that he must be bad because he has been treated badly. This ontological shift creates an awareness that we are not the center of the universe and our environment and relations with others inevitably shape us in positive and negative ways. However, pointing the finger of blame at the parents, one's first love objects or objects of attachment, gives rise to a sense of guilt often expressed in terms of, "How can I be angry at my parents who were only doing their best and were struggling themselves?" At this point, the patient is stuck in-between anger and guilt and may become despairing and/ or suicidal, directing their murderous feelings towards themselves. The very people who are to blame are those the patient depended on and who nourished him. The guilt at this stage is alleviated by the analyst's acknowledgement of the patient's anger, along with vengeful feelings, as legitimate. Once the patient feels free to acknowledge his own anger and hatred, he is then free to think about his predicament and how to live in the present. This is also a process in which the patient becomes acutely aware of how self-destructive his anger towards his parents has been, inadvertently causing hurt to others and himself. In seeing this, the patient becomes responsible for his own actions and can experience guilt for the damage he has caused. No one else can be blamed. It is at this point that the pain of one's destructive behavior and the losses that have been caused as a result, including the loss of innocence, can be truly felt. The only amelioration to this pain is the realization that increased self-awareness brings with it an increased ability to make choices in one's life and to accept responsibility and guilt when it is merited and not to revert to the narcissistic omnipotence of childhood guilt. Unless there is some acknowledgement on the part of the wrongdoer for the harm that has been done and some possibility of reconciliation,[11] the initial anger and blame towards those who have been hurtful never disappears. This does not mean, however, that the victim continues to be angry or to seek revenge; this merely perpetuates the victim's emotional attachment to the perpetrator. What it does mean is that the scars left have been recognized and accepted as such.

If we look at political conflict across the world we will quickly find that in many countries or groups that have experienced violent conflict over generations, even with attempts to resolve the conflict, there remain vendettas and anger towards the enemy that defy acceptance, much less resolution. Within large groups, blame towards others that have been hurtful does not disappear and cannot be worked through or accepted in the same way that is possible with individuals. Blame and virtue are memorialized respectively in the "chosen traumas" and "chosen glories" that hold the group together and at the same time prevent the group from evolving. Individuals can also hold onto grudges as well as victories but the consequences are not so wide-scale and devastating. While there are numerous examples of groups that change their political position and are able to mitigate or refrain from acting out violently, if group identity or the existence of the group is under too much threat, the group reverts to familiar defense patterns of demonizing the "other" and self-purification to consolidate its identity. Nations may learn from history but this does not necessarily lead to changes in human behavior. The Holocaust is an example, warning nations against committing genocide in the future, but it may serve as a more powerful warning never to be the victim – a position that paradoxically provokes enactment of violent behavior.

The psychoanalytic process of blame and acceptance I have described is not a smooth road; invariably there are bumps and wrong turnings on the way. It is also a process that occurs for most people, who may not have suffered such severe trauma and neglect, with ordinary maturation. In other words, it is a process that most of us have experienced and that continues to evolve within us as we mature and have greater insight into our pasts and ourselves. Despite our experience of how large groups behave, we nevertheless often imagine and expect large group behavior to mirror our individual experience and yet there is little actual evidence that collectively we are very good at processing our past and not repeating it. The post-Auschwitz warning, "never again", is at odds with the dictum "history repeats itself". While, for example, our awareness of the early warning signs of genocide may be greater and more sophisticated than they were in the past, we are still remarkably blind to their occurrence in the present. Because of our individual capacity to continue to develop emotionally, we can take responsibility for our actions and, even in the midst of disasters beyond our control, we can retain some view of life as a melioristic process of enrichment on an internal, intrapsychic level at the very least. If, however, we look at history, there is a glaring lack of emotional development when it comes to large group behavior; we want to believe, for example, that we are getting "better" at how we treat other humans and point to changes such as the legal abolition of slavery while turning a blind eye to other forms of slavery that occur daily in our world. We are still committing the atrocities we abhor in others, we are still scapegoating others for our social ills, we are still exploiting those less powerful than us, we are still wanting to show the world we are blameless, either by outright denial or gestures of atonement, and we are still confusing guilt with responsibility. As V.S. Naipaul's narrator in *A Bend in the River* observes, "The Europeans wanted gold and slaves, like everybody else; but at the same time they wanted statues put up to themselves as people who had done good things for the slaves" (Naipaul, 1980).

This discrepancy between individual and group behavior raises questions about how large groups function, how or whether large groups recover from trauma and in particular how they establish and reinforce their identity. In writing about group behavior, Wilfred Bion describes two basic group states of mind as exemplified by the Basic Assumption Group and the Work Group. Bion views groups in terms of serving a collective purpose for the survival of its members and to seek the truth. Recognizing reality, i.e. seeking the truth, is essential for group survival. Strangely, Bion does not discuss group identity and its importance in terms of group cohesion, the development of culture, and for actual survival. The "Basic Assumption" mentality is manifest when the group has been overwhelmed by powerful emotions:

> ... anxiety, fear, hate, love, hope, anger, guilt, depression (Bion, p. 166) – and has, as a result, lost touch with its purpose, and become caught up in an "unconscious group collusion" (Eisold, 2005b, p. 359); the outcome is "stagnation" (Bion, 1961, p.128).
>
> (French & Simpson, 2010, p.2)

Volkan describes a similar state that occurs in groups in which their identity – their way of life, their position in the world and their very existence – is threatened. The group then in fear seeks an omnipotent leader who will promise to rescue them and restore them to power *despite* the reality they face. This is patently evident in the recent wave of populist politics, fueled by autocratic leaders who support a return to the past as a way of defending against loss and, ultimately, extinction (Volkan, 2004).

Once the existence and identity of a large group is threatened, it experiences trauma. The reactions to this trauma are clear and consistent across different cultures and include various techniques of not only restoring power but cleansing the group of that which has threatened its existence. The recent takeover of Afghanistan by the Taliban is a clear example of a group, the Taliban, whose existence has been under threat for many years. In their struggle for survival, their politico-religious identity is paramount. The nonbelievers, the infidel, have to be either brought into the fold or extinguished. The "other" is demonized and blamed for the sins of the world – all that is destructive to Allah is located in the "other", establishing and reinforcing the purity of the group. This is a well-observed pattern of group behavior that is the primary motivator and instigator behind all aggressive military action. The history of Afghanistan, or any country that has been at war over any length of time, inevitably differs according to the lens through which it is viewed; Americans, Russians, Afghanis, British, create their own versions of history from their own perspectives. These are not simply records of what happened where and when, and who was involved, they are events that are imbued with moral judgements about right and wrong; who was victim and who was perpetrator. Most importantly, the trauma of the past remains alive in the present within all groups that have experienced violence.

While the particular memories within a group are acknowledged and "chosen" to constitute its history and, as such, establish the group's identity, this does not mean its version of history will be shared beyond the boundaries of the group itself. The "chosen" history of the group serves to consolidate its identity but it can also create a rigid defense against acknowledging any other possible interpretation of events, resulting in what Bion referred to as "stagnation". When a group's existence becomes too threatened, for example, and its identity and purpose is dependent on a single leader, then "stagnation" takes the form of a closed system. In this context, as we see in totalitarian states such as North Korea and China, perceptions and interpretations of the past, i.e. "history", are comprehensively shaped – and censored – to accord with the collective ideals of the group. The creation or re-creation of a group's history is inevitably determined by the self-image the group needs to promote to provide some illusion of security. The greater the threat to group identity, the more the group will revert to paranoid-schizoid ways of perceiving reality; this is when the group becomes most vulnerable to re-enacting past traumas embedded in the collective psyche.

In a discussion held in 2020 by the Nexus Institute, politicians and military commentators were asked, "Why don't we learn from history?" The consensus was that because we continue to have wars, we must "like" war. While this may seem to be a simplistic answer, it suggests that violent conflict serves an important role in group identity and in consolidating internal group cohesion. We define ourselves to a large extent in terms of who we are *not*, not simply who we are.

There is a strong argument, supported by sociologists such as Max Weber and Georg Simmel, and political scientists such as Michael Desch, that war is the most important factor in establishing "strong, centralized states and cohesive national polities" (Walt, 2016). The impetus to fight the enemy requires internal unity while it also promotes patriotism and the suppression of internal divisions. But as Simmel points out: "A group's complete victory over its enemies is ... not always fortunate ... Victory lowers the energy which guarantees the unity of the group; and the dissolving forces, which are always at work, gain hold" (Ibid.).

There are numerous examples of the drawbacks to victory and peace throughout history. Here are two brief examples. In Europe, e.g., the period from 1815 and the Treaty of Paris until the Crimean War of 1853 was relatively free from external threats. Yet during this same period there was an unprecedented breakdown in state cohesion and a series of internal upheavals across various European states. In the US, by 1850 external threats were inconsequential and yet by 1860 the American Civil War was about to erupt.

In contrast, the Cold War gave birth to the American federal state and strengthened national unity. Desch describes the Cold War as the "perfect type of threat" (Ibid.). It did not escalate to a state of war but it served to unify the states under threat and to enhance their alliance with one another. Since the end of the Cold War, the level of conflict in the world has generally been declining. While there is greater stability internally, this also allows for internal conflicts to surface and become more divisive. Desch argues, "The longer the period of reduced international security competition, the more likely are developed states to be plagued by the rise of narrow sectoral, rather than broad encompassing, interest groups" (Ibid.).

The lesson here is that reducing external dangers has a downside. Stephen Walt, Professor of International Relations at Harvard, argues:

> The less threatened we are by the outside world, the more prone we are to ugly quarrels at home. Even worse, peace may contain the seeds of its own destruction. As we are now seeing in the Middle East, the collapse of unity and state authority can easily trigger violent internal conflicts that eventually drag outside powers back in.
>
> (Ibid.)

If we accept the psychological advantages of war in relation to group identity and solidarity, then it would seem to follow that our repeated experiences of war or violent state conflict inevitably re-traumatize the groups involved. This in turn leads to further enactments of violence, strengthening collective trauma; whether as perpetrator or as victim, everyone has suffered.

Perhaps the most important difference between the individual and the group is the role that conflict plays in the formation of identity. While it is important in individual identity to be able to differentiate oneself from another, this is not the same thing as conflict. Although a small baby may experience his mother as all bad, in a paranoid state, this state will normally change once the baby is satisfied and it is safe once again to depend on the mother. Groups that have a relatively secure identity, even if short-lived, are in a better position to contain internal conflict but only until it reaches a tipping point when group cohesion is threatened.[12]

While individuals are dependent on the groups they belong to for their identity, groups are not in this position by their very nature. Countries depend on alliances with other countries but their identity – and their power – is founded on their separateness from other countries. This not only makes warfare more likely but the history of violence itself becomes a defining aspect of group identity.

As Freud wrote, the doctor "celebrates it as a triumph for the treatment if he can bring it about that something that the patient wishes to discharge in action is disposed of through the work of remembering" (Freud, 1958, p.153). When memory can be retrieved, there is no need to repeat the past. In relation to groups, however, this process is stymied because group identity is bound to and enmeshed with the group's history of trauma. Because of this the group cannot "remember" but can only respond in a binary way, pointing the finger of blame on to others. Bion's idea of "stagnation" applies here as the group identity is at stake when its "chosen history" is challenged. Through this lens of trauma, it is hardly surprising that groups are unable to experience guilt or other feelings based on a narrative they feel doesn't apply to them and when altering their "chosen history" threatens their very identity.

Conclusion

To reiterate Kohon's point, history "belongs to everyone and to no one" (Kohon, p.5). This is both its strength and its weakness. Because history is impersonal, it is susceptible to scrutiny and revision but it is also open to manipulation as it serves to preserve the identities of the groups that are its subject. Chosen traumas and chosen glories are important markers of past events that create face-saving narratives for the group in the present. The monuments and memorials of these chosen traumas/glories constitute a group's "chosen history" and, alongside this, a group's "chosen identity"; as such, their purpose is not to serve as complex icons to be learned from but, on the contrary, as proof of an immutable "truth" that is *not* subject to revision. They are the "facts", the traumas and the glories, literally set in stone. These same chosen traumas/glories then serve as a justification for enactments in their name.

Quite apart from the cohesive advantages of conflict, events such as the successive invasions of Afghanistan serve whichever national narrative of the chosen glory of whichever invading power is involved. The American invasion of Afghanistan soon took on the mantle of a national glory, spreading "freedom and democracy" to a subjugated people. This narrative is no different from every other imperial expansion in history that has been glorified in the name of some higher value. It is only when groups or nations fail that their failures become traumas and victors turn into victims, passing blame on to others. While as individuals we do have the ability to learn from our past and to understand that lessons from the past help us to survive, this is not evident in the case of groups, especially when they are threatened with extinction. Group identity is bolstered by its history of "chosen traumas" and "chosen glories" that in turn demand re-enactment to sustain the "truth". Trauma – and history – repeat themselves in a never-ending feedback loop.

In writing about the worldwide trend to erect grandiose memorials as significers of local history, the writer, Edwin Heathcote questions:

> Is it doing any good? The argument behind an architecture of permanence at this scale is a rejoinder not to forget. Yet it comes in parallel with a tsunami of misinformation and fake news spread through the fleetingly ephemeral digital media. The explosion of conspiracy theories, anti-science hokum, Holocaust denial and the rewriting of histories, both official and personal, is leading to a collapse in the narrative, an atomisation of national and cultural memory which even the grandest and weightiest of memorials are clearly failing to counter.
>
> The memorial that seems most poetic to me is not even there at all. Conceptual artist Jochen Gerz's Monument Against Fascism in Harburg, a suburb of Hamburg, is a lead-clad monolith on to which people were encouraged to scrawl and inscribe messages and names. It was lowered,

gradually, over years, until it disappeared beneath the ground, leaving only a small square of metal at the surface. Like memory, it is mostly buried, but it is always there.

(Heathcote, 2020)

Gerz's Monument symbolizes what has been lost, what is "not even there at all". In leaving only a trace of metal visible, the monument also symbolizes our buried violence, doomed to be forgotten but always there beneath the surface waiting to recur. Ultimately, we need to forget *and* remember the past in order to live anew in the present (Hyde, p.252).

Notes

1 I do not subscribe to the particular psychoanalytic view that there should be no goal to psychoanalytic treatment. Failure to acknowledge that there is a goal to this process is equivalent to denying our psychic need to develop and understand ourselves, our inner and external realities, and through this understanding not to be led blindly by the complexes of our past. Psychoanalysis is necessarily a teleological endeavour.

2 The importance placed on a group or nation's history reveals how it chooses to present itself to the world. In postwar and later in reunified Germany, for example, an honest appraisal of history after the end of the Third Reich was required as a way for the country to save face and to redeem itself in the eyes of the world. In contrast, for some time now the authorities in post-communist Russia have made it clear that there is no expectation or sense of moral obligation to Russian citizens to present a factual or honest account of the country's past, particularly with regard to the millions of lives lost under the repression of communist regimes. One example is the recent move taken by state prosecutors to shut down Memorial, a group founded in the 1980s to commemorate the victims of Soviet repression, in an attempt to erase this brutal period of history. Instead, a distorted narrative is created that allows the government to save face to its own citizens and to enhance its power both within Russia and abroad.

3 Since May 2018 Juvénal Habyarimana's villa, formerly the Presidential Palace Museum, has been renamed the Rwanda Art Museum.

4 Investigators from the International Criminal Tribunal for Rwanda point to Kagame as having given orders for Habyarimana's plane to be shot down. (See Rever, J., (11th October 2016). "Probe revisits mystery of assassination that triggered Rwandan genocide," *The Globe and Mail*.)

5 Alexievich notes, "The sheer volume of lies in our minds associated with Chernobyl bears comparison only with the situation at the outbreak of war in 1941 under Stalin." (Alexievich, 2016, p.185)

6 In her book, *The Punishment of Virtue* (2006), NPR correspondent Sarah Chayes argues: "I have often been asked whether we in the West have the right to 'impose democracy' on people who 'just might not want it,' or might not be 'ready for it.' I think, concerning Afghanistan at least, this question is exactly backward ... I have found that Afghans know precisely what democracy is—even if they might not be able to define the term. And they are crying out for it. They want from their government what most Americans and Europeans want from theirs: roads they can drive on, schools for their kids, doctors with certified qualifications ..., a minimum of public accountability, and security ... And they want to participate in some real way in the fashioning of their nation's destiny ... But Afghans were getting precious little of any of that ... American policy in Afghanistan was not imposing or

even encouraging democracy, as the US government claimed it was. Instead, it was standing in the way of democracy. It was institutionalizing violence." (In O'Toole, NYRB)

7 Groups such as the Roma and Sinti are often overlooked as Holocaust survivors signifying that they are not worthy of the rights and considerations accorded to other victim groups.

8 The exceptions are the leaders who have been caught out in corruption and must be expunged from the group to restore purity, the common examples being leaders who are threatened with impeachment.

9 Santayana actually wrote: "Those who cannot remember the past are condemned to repeat it." (Santayana, G., (1905). *The Life of Reason*, New York: Scribner) This statement has been typically understood as a warning not to forget the past, but it can equally be interpreted to mean that we repeat the past because we forget our history. I argue that it is not that history is forgotten but it is always manipulated and remembered to reinforce some narrative that ascribes national or group identity.

10 The misapplication of Judeo-Christian morality in political attempts to resolve or heal the trauma of collective violence is discussed in Chapter Six, "Rituals of Healing and the Perpetuation of Blame".

11 The possibility and meaning of reconciliation for large groups is discussed in Chapter Seven, "Rituals of Acknowledgement".

12 Inglehart and Norris argue convincingly that threats to group identity in the form, for example, of economic equality create instability and fear that lead to popularist authoritarian forms of leadership. (Norris, P. & Inglehart, R. (2019). *Cultural Backlash: Trump, Brexit, and Authoritarian Populism.* Cambridge: Cambridge University Press.)

References

Alexievich, S. (2016). *Chernobyl Prayer.* London: Penguin.

Bion, W.R. (1961). *Experiences in Groups.* London: Tavistock Publications.

French, R.B. & Simpson, P. (2010). "The 'work group': Redressing the balance in Bion's Experiences in Groups." *Human Relations*, 63(12), 1859–1878.

Freud, S. (1958)"Remembering, Repeating and Working-Through." In *The Standard Edition of the Complete Psychological Works of Sigmund Freud,* Vol. 12. Repr. 2001. London: Hogarth Press and the Institute of Psychoanalysis.

Heathcote, E. (15 December 2020). "Memorial rules and not set in stone." *Financial Times.*

Hyde, L. (2019). *A Primer for Forgetting: Getting Past the Past.* New York: Farrar, Straus & Giroux.

Kohon, G. (2021). "Monuments and denials: creating and re-creating history." *BPAS Bulletin.*

Mitton, K. (2015). *Rebels in a Rotten State: Understanding Atrocity in Sierra Leone.* London: Hurst & Co.

Naipaul, V.S. (1980). *A Bend in the River.* London: Penguin.

Nora, P. (1989). "Between memory and history: Les Lieux de Memoire." In *Representations, No. 26, Special Issue: Memory and Counter-Memory* (Spring, 1989), pp. 7–24. Oakland: University of California Press.

O'Toole, F. (7 October 2021). "The lie of nation building." *The New York Review of Books.*

Sebald, W.G. (2003). *On the Natural History of Destruction.* London: Hamish Hamilton.

Starritt, A. (2020). *We Germans*. London: JM Originals.

Subotić, J. (2019). *Yellow Star, Red Star*. Cornell: Cornell University Press.

Volkan, V. (2004). *Blind Trust: Large Groups and Their Leaders in Times of Crisis and Terror*. Charlottesville, Virginia: Pitchstone Publishing.

Walt, S.M. (17 June 2016). "The Case Against Peace." *Foreign Policy*.

Wrong, M. (27 April 2016). "The False Idols of Rwanda's Genocide." *Foreign Policy*.

Chapter 6

Rituals of Healing and the Perpetuation of Blame

Even revenge doesn't really work.

(Anna, rape victim)

In the aftermath of large-scale violence most cultures turn to traditional rituals or create new ones to heal the wounds of traumatized communities. Judeo-Christian cultures place particular emphasis on guilt, forgiveness and atonement. These rituals are meant to restore moral order, to cleanse the group of shame and hatred and to establish a common narrative or memory of what has happened. They are also meant to prevent or bring to a close cycles of vengeance and differ in this respect to forms of retributive justice that impose punishment. The problem with this moral tradition and the problem underlying ritualized attempts to restore peace between perpetrators and victims is that they are largely based on a binary understanding of good and evil, right and wrong, victims and offenders, and are concerned with restoring social equity for an aggrieved group. The finger of blame is pointed and yet true healing is meant to eradicate blame. This inherent contradiction contains the seeds of failure. Rather than helping to contain and mitigate conflict within a group, this approach runs the risk of creating further psychological splitting, delineating an us-them opposition even more sharply and establishing a moral high ground that reinforces political superiority. The other problem with this approach to peace-making is that it treats large groups as if they are individuals acting as if prompted by a single will and as if they were a single agency. While a nation's identity is central to its survival, this does not mean that there is a national or collective psyche that experiences trauma in the same way that an individual does. "Psychologizing the nation" can be helpful in understanding political dynamics but is unhelpful when we transpose individual responses to trauma to group behavior. The rituals intended to restore peace and heal national trauma, because they are founded on the premise that groups behave like individuals, either perpetuate a culture of blame or have little effect on it. Individual participants may benefit but wide-scale conflict cannot be resolved.

DOI: 10.4324/9781003379980-7

Who is to Blame?

The central question that underlies any attempt to adjudicate and heal large-scale violence is whom to hold responsible and how to weigh individual responsibility within a group. The problem of distinguishing between collective and individual guilt first arose in international legal jurisprudence in the formation of the Nuremberg Trials. The Allies debated at length about how to deliver retributive justice against the Germans who had committed atrocities and damage to other countries on such a large scale. Initially, the British leaders and many American politicians called for the summary execution of Nazi leaders, following military tradition. The Russians, however, called for an international tribunal that would bring world attention to the concept of war as "a crime against peace". This idea was introduced by the Russian lawyer, Aron Trainin, who described "the planning and waging of an unprovoked war of conquest as a punishable criminal act" (Hirsch, 2020, p.8). Trainin's seminal proposal provided the cornerstone for the trials, paving the way for the concept of crimes against humanity and genocide that later evolved. From the Soviet point of view, Trainin's proposal was also welcome in diverting attention away from Soviet crimes committed during the war and promoted the image of communism as concerned with higher forms of social justice. Along with the idea of collective guilt, Trainin introduced ideas about complicity and criminal responsibility pertaining to individual members of what were recognized to be "criminal" groups. In this way, Trainin was trying to identify and hold accountable "criminal groups" that had been instrumental in leading and enforcing Nazi rule and to challenge the common defense amongst individual members that they were simply following orders. These nuanced degrees of responsibility and guilt highlighted the complexity of differentiating between collective and individual guilt that remain inextricably linked. In recognizing the concept of collective guilt within international law, the Nuremberg Trials gave birth to the concept of collective justice and collective forms of healing, and to the misapprehension that collective entities can be equated to individuals in terms of responsibility, moral intent and emotional processes such as mourning, guilt and forgiveness.

This confusion between individual and group responsibility is evident in the practice of the International Criminal Court that has the power to bring to trial individual leaders of countries or large groups (e.g. militia) accused of committing atrocities, including acts of genocide. While this may be the only pragmatic way of instituting some form of retributive justice, it often leaves the perpetrator regime intact or becomes a means for a new regime to absolve itself of past crimes. While nations are increasingly expected to accept responsibility for their "crimes", it is individuals who are ultimately held to account and, as such, become stand-ins for the group; their punishment or elimination cleanses the group of its misdeeds.[1]

Although every group has its own rituals for dealing with miscreant individual members in order to restore the social and moral order within the group, these are primarily at an individual level and do not normally encompass large groups that have been engaged in violence. In these cases, conflict between large groups has traditionally been resolved or has ceased through mutual agreement such as war treaties. Resolution or an agreement to cease fighting, however, does not mean that the conflict has gone away or will not rear its head again in time. It was the Holocaust and the way in which retribution and justice were applied that planted the seeds of future attempts at peace-making and reparation on a collective basis. The proliferation of truth and reconciliation commissions since the first truth commissions were established in South America in the 1980s, followed by the South African Truth and Reconciliation Commission in 1995, testify to the hope that establishing a collective narrative or truth and bringing together victims and offenders will create a healing process that ensures longer lasting peace for the future. While many of these commissions have been beneficial for individual victims, there is no substantial research on their effect on perpetrators. In terms of political impact, they have largely failed in healing the traumas that inevitably remain in the collective memory and are only too easily repeated in the present.

Truth and Justice

Individuals who have been traumatized want to know why this has happened to them and why the perpetrators did what they did; they also want the injustice of their suffering to be acknowledged and put right. In the private context of psychoanalysis, the key factor in the healing process is establishing and validating the "truth". The analyst performs the function of witness and, in this role, verifies the psychic reality of the patient, establishing that the patient was hurt and traumatized in reality and, even in the face of necessarily incomplete and unreliable memory, the effects of the trauma are real and have created layers of damage, including self-harm. Understanding the source of inner conflict and being able to restore trust in one's perceptions and judgment enables the traumatized patient to separate and recover from the taint of being treated as an object and from the self-hatred that accompanies this. Truth in this context incorporates a reconstruction of the actual harm that has been inflicted, sometimes over long periods of time, alongside the truth of how the patient has perceived these events and made sense of them to create some narrative that will make sense of something that is otherwise incomprehensible. Truth becomes both personal and public (i.e. witnessed) and in the process of reconstruction both analyst and patient accept that the narrative and the truth that it conveys will inevitably change and become more nuanced.

The truth commissions were initially set up in South America in the 1980s as a means of implementing transitional justice[2] and establishing public trust in new civilian governments that had supplanted military regimes. Since this time, over forty countries have embarked on truth commissions ranging widely in their scope and aims. In the case of addressing the disappearance of individuals in Argentina and Chile under repressive regimes, these commissions helped to verify the deaths of individuals and in some instances how the murders had been committed, but did not, on the whole, attempt to address why this had happened. Michael Ignatieff, in his seminal paper, "Articles of Faith", comments:

> One should distinguish between factual truth and moral truth, between narratives that tell what happened and narratives that attempt to explain why things happened and who is responsible. The truth commissions were more successful in promoting the first than the second. They did succeed in establishing the facts about the disappearance, torture and death of thousands of persons and this allowed relatives and friends the consolation of knowing how the disappeared had met their fate. It says much for the human need for truth that the relatives of victims preferred the moral appeal of magnanimity that so many of them should have preferred the truth to vengeance or even justice. It was sufficient for them to know what happened: they did not need to punish the transgressors in order to put the past behind them.
>
> The record of the truth commissions in Latin America has however disillusioned many of those who believed that shared truth was a precondition of social reconciliation. The military and police apparatus survived the inquisition with their legitimacy undermined but their power intact.
>
> (Ignatieff, 1996)

Ignatieff goes on to point out that the truth commissions did not in fact set out to create social reconciliation[3]; they were not mandated to change institutional structures or to implement social reform. As Ignatieff emphasizes, truth by itself cannot do this. Nor can truth guarantee or lead to justice. The most important healing factor for the victims' families and friends was in knowing what had happened. Here, what is true is factual truth and, as in the case of an individual patient, having this "truth" acknowledged enables the victims to re-inhabit a reality that is not always in question and in this way to separate from a past full of what is unknown and unthinkable. But Ignatieff also points out that factual or sequential, narrative truth is different from moral truth, i.e. how violence is understood, who has responsibility for what and, most importantly, who is to blame. Moral truth-seeking attempts to regain a sense of control in what has become a morally disordered universe (Rock, 1998). Reconciliation requires shared moral or interpretive truth and, as we see in countries around the world, this is rare indeed. Even in those countries that accept responsibility and blame, as Germany has for the atrocities committed during World War Two, the shared moral truth that has been constructed is complex and invariably masks other versions of the truth that may not be overtly politically acceptable but emerge, like the repressed, in other forms in the political arena.

Referring to the Balkans, Ignatieff raises the improbability of Serbians and Croatians ever agreeing on who is to blame. The truth of each group lies in its own history of grievances and triumphs, in its chosen glories and chosen traumas; these constitute group identity. As Ignatieff notes:

> Peoples who believe themselves to be victims of aggression have an understandable incapacity to believe that they also committed atrocities. Myths of innocence and victimhood are a powerful obstacle in the way of confronting unwelcome facts.
>
> (Ignatieff, 1996)

If we look at civil wars or nations with long-standing histories of conflict, they may be able to reach some form of agreed or controlled peace but, as in Rwanda, Palestine and Israel, South Africa, Sierra Leone, Sri Lanka, and so on, the grievances of the past remain in the present, like Gerz's Monument, buried but alive beneath the surface. Traumas do not go away for either the individual or the group. Here again we face the conundrum of trying to resolve large group conflicts by means of establishing social and psychological processes for individual victims and perpetrators who cannot represent the larger group. It is a category error, similar to expecting a dysfunctional family to change because one of its members has had therapy. Unless the group is able to recognize its own destructiveness, nothing will change. For nations whose identity is founded on what I have called a chosen narrative or history, we may be expecting a leopard to change its spots.

Forgiveness and Reconciliation

While establishing factual truth is of primary importance to our lives in validating our perception of reality, most of us aspire to peaceful coexistence and the resolution of conflict, or at the very least a state of truce. Within Western Judeo-Christian tradition, resolution of conflict is often seen to be dependent on the capacity for forgiveness, as if the act of forgiveness will turn a new page and restore equity or balance between enemies alongside social order. However, true forgiveness requires a mutual recognition of wrongdoing; the offender must apologize. Without this, forgiveness is meaningless at best and at worst a form of denial or self-righteous superiority.[4] Although Christianity urges us to forgive our enemies, in Catholic doctrine only God has the power to confer forgiveness as any sin is ultimately one against God. In the New Testament, some sins, such as sins against children, remain beyond forgiveness.[5] In the face of these limits of forgiveness, it is nevertheless emphasized as a desirable predicator of peace and points more to our human desire to believe that we have the power to forgive our enemies, regardless of their consent, and to purify and mend the damaged fabric of social relations. We want to believe there is a solution that will transcend memory and history.

The expression, "Forgive, but never forget", warns us that forgiveness, whether or not it is even possible, has its dangers. In an interview on Yad Vashem and the possibility of forgiveness, the French philosopher, Jacques Derrida, makes it clear that pure forgiveness for the Holocaust is impossible, both for those who survived and their descendants who may nevertheless find it easier to reconcile and to mourn because they were not its immediate victims. Derrida warns that our desire to preserve memory, as in the Yad Vashem archives, contains the seeds for forgetting as it strips memory of its emotional content. It becomes an artefact rather than a lived experience. He explains:

> ... it is the very act of archivizing which contributes somehow to classification, relativization and forgetting. Archivization preserves, but it also begins to forget. And it is possible that one day, and one thinks of this with horror, Yad Vashem will be considered as just another monument. Because it is kept, consigned to the exteriority of archives, because it is here between walls, everything has been recorded, a CD Rom was made, the names are on plaques, and so because it is kept, well, it may be lost, it may be forgotten. There is always this risk, and that is the ambiguity of the concept of archive, that I've been concerned with elsewhere, one always runs the risk of losing (what) one keeps and of forgetting precisely where memory is objectivized in acts of consignment, in objective places.
>
> (Derrida, 1998, interview)

Just as Derrida reassigns memory to individual experience, he also emphasizes that forgiveness, if it is at all possible, is a personal choice and act, implying that once it becomes a collective imperative or a collective act, it assumes a moral valance that is antithetical to the meaning of forgiveness. Derrida continues:

> Having said this, your question was: "should one forgive after Auschwitz?" I'd say that in no case does anyone have the right to say one should forgive or one should not forgive ... (P)ure or unconditional forgiveness must be the event or the act of a grace that cannot be commanded. There shouldn't be a duty to forgive or a duty not to forgive. In other words, if pure forgiveness, with regard to Auschwitz or anything whatever, is to take place, it is for each person to come to it, to take responsibility for it in a unique way without entering into any economy of judgement, of penalty, of punishment, etc. Forgiveness is within our domain; this is why I distinguished forgiveness from limitation, from limitability. I don't believe that the experience of forgiveness, if such there

be, can lend itself to judgements of the order of: "Now one must forgive", or: "One must not forgive". The question of limitation, the legal, political question is quite different from the question of forgiveness. But as to forgiveness, only the victims have the right to forgive. Forgive whom, actually? Who forgives whom? It would be up to the victims themselves to forgive or not forgive the butchers. But we are today the heirs of the victims or the heirs of the butchers. And the question of forgiveness cannot be asked today as such, in pure form.

(Derrida, interview)

Although Derrida suggests the impossibility of forgiveness as it pertains to any group, the appeal of many of the truth and reconciliation commissions has been that not only are they intended to create a collective narrative of events, a shared truth that is recounted and agreed upon publicly, but that this narrative can then be "remembered" collectively and not forgotten. Inevitably, the "truth" that is established reflects the way in which events are interpreted and given meaning. The public testimony of victims and perpetrators is intended to provide a path towards forgiveness; above all this is dependent on perpetrators acknowledging the harm they have inflicted.

The promise of achieving lasting reconciliation rests on the two corner-stones of shared memory and forgiveness. In the framework of the South African Truth and Reconciliation Commission, what was sought was not retributive justice but restorative justice – a concept that has formed the basis of subsequent truth and reconciliation commissions and purports to be a form of social healing. The powerful appeal of restorative justice is that it promotes the illusion that what has been lost or broken can be restored. In reality this is a promise that cannot be fulfilled because the loss can never be remedied. The concept of restoration in itself suggests that the past, however it is imagined, represents a desirable state to return to; it does not address pre-existing conflicts or the structural issues at the heart of violence.

Archbishop Tutu likened the reconciliation process to the African concept of *ubuntu* that emphasizes human equality and connectedness, summarized as "a person is a person through other people", in which social relationships assume greater importance than exacting vengeance on the perpetrator. The idea of *ubuntu*, however, derives its strength from communities in which there is already some form of social cohesion or connectedness, in which the fabric of social relations is of paramount importance. In such communities, rituals of purification and reincorporation of the individual perpetrator/offender are often vital in maintaining group identity. But this does not apply in the case of opposing groups or large group animosity. While the principle of *ubuntu* may work well in individual instances, its effectiveness in reconciliation is questionable precisely because the perpetrators' position is not given recognition from the start and therefore real equity is never established.

The main difficulty conceptually in the political concept and practice of reconciliation is that it confuses individual psychological processes with group processes and confuses a discourse of justice with what may be described as "a language of therapy and healing, or the moral and religious discourse of forgiveness" (Avruch, 2002, p.41). Not only are notions of punishment and retribution lost in this process, but, ironically, so is the notion of equity – for both the individual victim and for the perpetrator. In their review of truth and reconciliation commissions, Kevin Avruch and Beatriz Vejarano, point out:

> ... it is precisely in trying to apply what may be therapeutically effective at the interpersonal level to the collective level that reconciliation often seems to lose clarity and become more ambiguous as an approach to peacebuilding. Can we talk about individual healing in the same breath as national healing? How exactly is the shift from the individual to the societal going to be brought about? Lerche (2000), Goodman (1999), Ignatieff (1996) evince some skepticism here, while Tutu (2000), Lederach (1999), and Montville (n.d.) are more hopeful. In an interesting analysis of the South African case, Wilson (2000) underlines the value inherent in recognizing individual suffering and collectivizing it, as the South African TRC did through its televised hearings. A new political identity was constructed, that of "national victim". In this way, individual suffering was brought into a public space to be shared by all, "made sacred in order to construct a new national collective conscience". In contrast, Winslow (1997) argues that while the South African TRC has worked in some ways to affect reconciliation at the collective level, this can occur at the expense of individual, psychological healing. Healing at the individual level is independent of collective reconciliation.
>
> (Avruch, p.41)

One of the sharpest criticisms of the South African Truth and Reconciliation Commission and other subsequent commissions is that they delivered "victor's justice" in the sense of condemning those perceived as the perpetrators or criminals. Reconciliation tends to be based on a formula of acknowledgement and contrition from the perpetrators and forgiveness from the victims. In this way, both victim and offender are reified in a paranoid-schizoid identification and the notion of equity is lost. The traditional colonial split between us and them continues to be mirrored in the tribunals in reforming the same narrative of oppressors and oppressed. This process of vilification of the enemy is not only an attempt to regain a collective morality demarcating right from wrong but also to purify the group from the threat of internal destructiveness by projecting this onto others. Such splitting is also a natural defense against trauma but will result in repeated narratives of violence if it remains unintegrated. We can see this happening typically in instances of intransigent political conflict in which both sides project their own aggression onto the other and so perpetuate fear and continual attack in the name of self-defense.

It is striking that, while reconciliation processes provide a forum for victims to give voice to their suffering and for their experience to be witnessed and validated, we rarely come across any accounts from the perpetrators who are largely seen as in the wrong, if not evil, with little attempt at understanding their position.[6] The political scientist, Kieran Mitton, comments that in the case of Sierra Leone, victims' outrage did not produce guilt or shame in the perpetrators but led to greater schism and resentment:

> Perversely, the moral outrage of victims of violence may in itself have provoked moral outrage from their tormentors. In this sense, it was not that victims stirred up dormant or deeply-buried feelings of guilt or shame in perpetrators, but that perpetrators felt angry that actions that were morally justified and celebrated within the rebel world were being condemned. Combined with anger over perceived civilian betrayal, this may account for the discomforting "genuine sense of outrage and self-righteousness" that Keen observed among many young Sierra Leonean fighters (Keen, 2012a:204).
>
> (Mitton, 2015, pp.159–60)

This sense of outrage amongst perpetrators, often silenced or repressed, can act as a tinder box for future conflict and violence.

Reparation

Another form of healing conflict that is used on its own or in conjunction with rituals of reconciliation is reparation in which the perpetrators, as part of an attempt to restore social equity, offer reparation to the victims usually in the form of financial reparation, restoration of property or repatriation. The act of reparation on the part of nations is perhaps most important in acknowledging the injustice that has been inflicted on a persecuted group and as an attempt to right this wrong. It is, however, also fraught with problems on several levels, such as the timeframe taken into account, the amount and form of reparation considered appropriate and the effect of reparation on victims. These different forms of reparation constitute symbolic acts on the part of the government that recognize injustice and, notwithstanding the importance of public acknowledgement, they do not absolve and in fact may exacerbate blame, especially when victims view reparation as a means of being bought off. Here again, there tends to be a confusion between addressing individual victims and a class of victims. Individual responses to reparation varies with some victims feeling that justice has been served, others that no money can restore what has been lost, and still others viewing it as a form of inauthentic closure that relieves the perpetrator from further responsibility.

The recurring cry for financial reparation to descendants of slaves in the US and elsewhere is an example of some of the limitations of reparation as a form of restoring justice or equity in a society riven with inequities at every social level.

Similarly, while restoring stolen property (whether it is land or valuable objects) to victims may be seen as an important act intended to reverse harm done and, as such, of benefit to many individual victims, it has little effect on victims as a group and the many other forms of loss that they have suffered. Perhaps the most effective act of reparation that we have seen instituted by any government is the offer of repatriation. This is notably the case in Germany where, since 20th August 2021, under Article 116 par.2 of the Basic Law (*Grundgesetz*), legal provision is made for victims of Nazi persecution forced to leave the country for political, racial or religious grounds between 30th January 1933 and 8th May 1945 and for their descendants to apply for restoration of their citizenship. For individual victims, this provision undoubtedly has a profound impact on their lives[7] and reinstates belonging to the group in a way which other forms of reconciliation cannot achieve. Repatriation has the ability to incorporate the group of victims back into the larger group, transforming their identity from victim to member. Through this process the group is able not only to be reincorporated but they are able to re-identify as Germans.

Reintegration: the Case of Rwanda

Violent conflict permeates large groups with hatred, instability, lack of trust, paranoid relationships – all the effects of trauma that threaten to disable healthy functioning and to destroy social cohesion. Strategies to heal the traumatic effects of conflict, such as reconciliation and reparation, are aimed at upholding concepts of justice in terms of recognition of crimes committed but go further in their attempt to mend social divisions caused by conflict. Some of the conceptual and methodological pitfalls of these strategies are illustrated in the case of post-genocide Rwanda.

Following the 1994 genocide in Rwanda, President Kagame and his government recognized the need to bring opposing groups together in order to heal its traumatic past and to prevent future hostilities. While economic progress within the country has been remarkable, it has also been clear that its future stability relies on the integration of Rwandan society post-conflict. The government drew on its indigenous traditions of peace-making to promote social cohesion in the form of three social innovations: *gacaca, ingando* and *umushyikirano.*

Gacaca is a form of community justice that combines elements of both retributive and restorative justice, establishing both punishment and reconciliation as its goal. Initiated in 2002 as a social experiment to redress at a local level some of the crimes committed during the genocide, it has been highly criticized on a number of grounds and its effectiveness seems to have been limited. Many of the criticisms reflect similar criticisms aimed at the South African Truth and Reconciliation Commission. The most important criticisms are enumerated by Omar McDoom in his World Development Report 2011 on Rwanda. These are:

> (i) Gacaca is victor's justice: War crimes have been explicitly excluded from the competence of gacaca courts, thus leaving allegations of RPF (Rwandan Patriotic Front) crimes committed during the civil war and genocide unaddressed in the minds of the Hutu community; (ii) Gacaca does not offer proper redress for victims of sexual violence: Given the stigma attached to such crimes for the victims, fewer have been reported to the community than have occurred; (iii) Gacaca has limited support from the population: Gacaca courts have suffered from low participation levels from the community, and the need for the state to enforce attendance from above has raised questions of to what extent restorative justice is being fulfilled and to what extent gacaca could be fairly described as a local, customary institution; (iv) Gacaca has led to the perversion of justice: While we do not have systematic evidence of how widespread the problems are, research has suggested that false accusations have been made to settle personal scores, false confessions made to receive lower sentences, witnesses intimidated, and deals struck leading to the acquittal of guilty individuals; (v) Gacaca does not provide restitution: Survivors of the genocide feel inadequately compensated for their loss and suffering.
>
> (McDoom, 2011, p.18)

McDoom points out that some of these criticisms could have been resolved through reform and greater government enforcement. Its strength – and what distinguished it from the Truth and Reconciliation Commission – is that it brings survivors and perpetrators together on a local level. This does not, however, necessarily ensure a better outcome. What is clearly evident is that the local resolution of conflicts and restoration of justice is only as good as the local political structure and the leaders who operate within that structure.

The second tradition of *ingando* was specifically intended to promote inter-ethnic reconciliation and national unity in Rwanda. *Ingando* was an educative process that brings Rwandans together to live in "solidarity camps" of up to a hundred residents for periods of several days to several weeks. It provides a safe space in which differences of views, history, and continuing conflicts can be brought out and potentially resolved. McDoom observes that *ingando*

> could encourage Rwandans to think independently and critically about their past. If Rwandans are instead trained to accept there is a single narrative which comes from the "high authorities", there is nothing to stop another government from teaching them something different (and

more dangerous) in the future. For example, ingando today emphasizes that Hutu and Tutsi co-existed happily until the advent of colonialism when the Belgians set them against each other. In contrast, the narrative taught in schools before the genocide was that Tutsi had historically oppressed Hutu and that they were alien to Rwanda. In the absence of critical thinking, a different government could in principle re-instill such a narrative of Rwanda's past.

(McDoom, p.20)

Like with *gacaca*, the process of *ingando* is only as effectives as the leaders who are behind it.[8]

The third innovation is that of *umushyikirano*, Rwanda's annual National Dialogue. *Umushyikirano* was also inaugurated in 2002 to provide a two-day national conference in which several hundred key Rwandan leaders from different sectors of society come together for public debate and dialogue. Much like its local counterpart, the *ingando, umushyikirano* also relied on providing a safe space in which conflict can be expressed and thought about, especially important in relation to the ethnic divisions that continue to beset Rwandan society. While this has been an important initiative, it is again only as effective as the political structure within which it operates. Accounts of Kagame's autocratic control over dissident factions and press reporting within Rwanda have only just begun to come into public view within the last few years.[9] Without freedom of the press and freedom of political parties, it is difficult to regard these processes as anything but perverse forms of smoothing over social conflicts that are in fact continuing to be repressed. As with many other countries trying to rid themselves of unseemly pasts, public relations are used as the means to purify and sanctify the new regimes.

There is, however, also a conceptual problem about these more local strategies of social reintegration within communities. They depend on two assumptions, the first being that communities were integrated prior to the genocide, and the second being that local communities operate on relatively self-sufficient lines. As McDoom points out, conflict between Hutus and Tutsis is long standing and, due to its history of violence, easily rekindled as the genocide proved. The second assumption relies on the belief that localized approaches to restoring justice are more effective than national approaches in empowering citizens to address directly their local conflicts. Traditional forms of community justice and ritual healing generally aim to mark out and punish the offender and then to perform ritual acts of reintegration, bringing the offender back within the group and its norms. The typical pattern is to expel the offender from the community for a period of time so as to purify the group and to then reintegrate the offender through ritualized acceptance. The success of this process depends on the fact that within small communities, expulsion is paramount to death, and reintegration is essential to continue to live. This is not the case, however, within larger communities in which interdependencies are more complex and in which oppositional divisions are likely to exist.

A further problem is in the nature of the crime committed; if the crime is outside the bounds of normative behavior within the group, such as genocide, customary remedies hardly apply. Apart from the fact that the these traditional local forms of restorative justice were not set up to address the scale and extremity of mass-killing, the trauma experienced by the entire community is in itself incapacitating, leaving the population in a kind of social limbo, lacking trust in its leaders and bewildered by the apparent ease at which social norms could be perverted and dismissed altogether.

In his analysis of these traditional restorative approaches, McDoom emphasizes that they are only as good as the leaders and the central government that support them. This is nevertheless a risky presumption because it assumes that, under capable and honest guidance, the resolution of national conflicts can be achieved at a local, individual level. This was particularly true in the case of the *gacaca* courts and the *ingando* education camps. What these processes overlook is that group identity is rarely homogeneous and is not transformed so easily; while some individuals may benefit, this does not mean that the group will or that reconciliation between groups will be anything more than lip service. The tradition of *umushyikirano* stands apart somewhat from the others insofar as it provides a pathway for communication between leaders of different groups. Pathways such as this do not, as we know, necessarily result in healing but they can establish a level playing field at best of mutual respect and recognition – but only if both sides are treated equally, and in post-genocide situations this is extremely unlikely if not perhaps impossible.[10]

Revenge

Revenge tends to be a dirty word within Judeo-Christian morality – we are applauded as virtuous when we forgive and condemned as brutish and mindless if we seek revenge. And yet, who does not want revenge when they or their families and loved ones have been killed or badly hurt? Retributive justice offers a measure of revenge in terms of punishing the wrongdoer. For many individual victims, this is sufficient revenge and, as such, enables them to separate emotionally from the perpetrator. In my experience of working with individual patients, even when their grievance against, for example, the parent who hurt them is validated, what continues to keep them attached to a relationship of pain is the wish for revenge, a revenge that is not actually possible for whatever reason. Blame and grievance remain after any injury but the drive for revenge can only be mitigated if it is satisfied in some way. The perpetrator who "gets away with it" remains a thorn in the side of his victim forever.

Brandon Hamber and Richard Wilson point out that wanting to avenge the death of a loved one is not motivated by sadism but is a "way of respecting the person who has died, to make their death and memory meaningful" (Hamber & Wilson, 2010, p.47). In *The Warrior's Honor*, Ignatieff asserts that the lasting hold of revenge over people's lives is misunderstood.

> Ignatieff recognizes that revenge is a profound moral desire to keep faith with the dead, to honour their memory by taking up their cause where they left off. To this end, revenge keeps faith between generations and the violence that follows is a ritual form of respect for the community's dead. For Ignatieff, therein lies the legitimacy of revenge.
>
> (Ibid.)

The need for revenge is not only out of respect for the deceased, it is also fundamental in restoring respect for the survivors. Injustice is being left in a position of humiliation and non-existence, as an object that has no agency. Erich Fromm views revenge as a kind of "magical reparation" that expunges or cancels out the perpetrator's crime; it is an act that restores self-agency (Fromm, 1984). Within the context of a group, revenge becomes an important aspect of protecting and preserving the group's identity, not just its self-respect but its ability to survive external threats. Although processes of reconciliation and reparation attempt to restore a sense of justice in relation to recalibrating a more equal position between victims and perpetrators, they cannot reverse the lack of self-agency that is promised by revenge, nor can they reinforce group identity so fundamentally. The obvious problem is that revenge feeds on itself in a timeless cycle that perpetuates blame. As Machiavelli warns, "Never do any enemy a small injury for they are like a snake which is half beaten and it will strike back the first chance it gets" (Machiavelli, 1513, Chapter 3, n.p.).

Notes

1 In trying to understand how evil comes about, the immediate common explanation is that it is because of an evil leader. This places responsibility on the leader alone while exonerating the group and the culture that chooses, supports and complies with a perverse regime. The problem of how to deal with collective evil both on a philosophical and practical level remains.

2 "Transitional justice" refers to public platforms set up in the aftermath of brutal regimes to establish the truth, to hold perpetrators to account, to allow victims to voice their grievances, to compensate victims and to enable a transition to law and order and institutional reforms under new government.

3 Truth commissions have been considered more effective if they are undertaken within a broader system of transitional justice and incorporate criminal proceedings, reparations, and systemic structural reform. However, even in these cases, the benefits for individual victims are not always evident and may even be detrimental, and there is no evidence they have an effect on group attitudes or behavior.

4 For a full discussion of the concept of forgiveness see "The problem of forgiveness and reparation in the aftermath of evil", Chapter Seven in Covington, C. (2017). *Everyday Evils: A Psychoanalytic View of Evil and Morality*. London: Routledge.

5 Luke, in the Gospels, declares, "It were better for him that a millstone were hanged about his neck, and he cast into the sea, than that he should offend one of these little ones." (Luke, 17,2)
6 In a landmark International Criminal Court trial in 2016, the Ugandan commander of the Lord's Resistance Army, Dominic Ongwen, pleaded not guilty of committing atrocities on the grounds that he had been abducted at the age of ten by the LRA and forced to become a child soldier. Ongwen claimed he was not a perpetrator, but a victim.
7 See my account of Sophie in Chapter Four of Covington, C., (2021) *For Goodness Sake: Bravery, Patriotism and Identity*, Phoenix Publishing House.
8 *Gacaca* courts ceased to operate along with the International Criminal Tribunal in Arusha that was dissolved in 2016. Sixty-one individuals were tried under the ICTR, not one of whom was a member of Rwanda Patriotic Front.
9 See Wrong, M. (2021). *Do Not Disturb: The Story of a Political Murder and an African Regime Gone Bad*. London: 4th Estate.
10 In the case of Northern Ireland, it was only by literally sharing the same table on an equal basis that the Northern Ireland Peace Talks achieved what they did.

References

Avruch, K. & Vejarano, B. (2002). "Truth and Reconciliation Commissions: A Review Essay and Annotated Bibliography." *The Online Journal of Peace and Conflict Resolution* 4(2), pp. 37–76.
Derrida, J. (8 January 1998). "Interview With Professor Jacques Derrida, Ecole des Hautes Etudes en Sciences Sociales, Paris." *Yad Vashem.*
Ferrari, J. (2010). *Where I Left My Soul.* London: Maclehose Press, Quercus.
Fromm, E. (1984). *The Anatomy of Human Destructiveness.* Harmondsworth: Penguin.
Hamber, B. & Wilson, R.A. (3 August 2010). "Symbolic closure through memory, reparation, and revenge in post-conflict societies." *Journal of Human Rights* 1(1), pp. 35–53.
Hirsch, F. (2020). *Soviet Judgment at Nuremberg: A New History of the International Military Tribunal after World War II.* Oxford: Oxford University Press.
Ignatieff, M. (September 1996). "*Articles of Faith.*" *Index on Censorship*, 5(96).
Ignatieff, M. (1998). *The Warrior's Honor: Ethnic War and the Modern Conscience.* London: Chatto & Windus.
Machiavelli, N. (1513) (2009). *The Prince.* London: Penguin.
McDoom, O. (2011). "Rwanda's Exit Pathway from Violence: A Strategic Assessment. World Development Report 2011: Background Paper." Washington DC: World Bank.
Mitton, K. (2015). *Rebels in a Rotten State: Understanding Atrocity in Sierra Leone.* London: Hurst & Company.
Rock, P. (1998). *After Homicide: Practical and Political Responses to Bereavement.* London: Clarendon Press.

Chapter 7

The Myth of Closure

In the end, we never get over anything.

(Maria, political exile)

Our human reaction to violence of any kind is to try by whatever means we can to cancel it out, to erase it, to be forgiven, to forget it, or alternatively to avenge it, to have it acknowledged, to be compensated, and to be reconciled. But perhaps most important is the wish to recover and to put the violence behind us, to put it in the past, to have it done with, to come to peace with it. The healing rituals examined in the previous chapter, such as truth and reconciliation commissions, restorative justice processes and reparation, are all attempts to produce closure on violent events so that they are not repeated in the future. As we have seen, these rituals may be effective for some of the individuals involved but have not proven to be effective on a political level or as a stopgap to further conflict. They are fraught with problems, largely derived from proscriptive religious beliefs that determine how we *ought* to behave, what we *ought* to believe and how we *ought* to banish hatred from our lives. These good intentions have failed spectacularly and yet we continue to believe we can change just as we continue to look for ways to create closure.

Mourning

In countries where there is a history of political violence and trauma that continues to repeat itself, one common explanation for this repetition is that the collective has not been able to mourn the violence of the past and, because of this and experiences that cannot be thought about or made sense of, the collective identifies with the aggressor and the cycle of violence is perpetuated. The assumption is that the collective can only heal itself from the violence it has experienced through the process of mourning, including acknowledgment of guilt and forgiveness from those who have been harmed. There is, however, a double confusion that underlies this assumption: the first confusion, as we have seen in other models of healing, is that group processes are identical to individual psychological behavior; the second confusion is

DOI: 10.4324/9781003379980-8

that loss and trauma can be treated similarly and overcome equally. These misconceptions lie at the heart of why mourning on a collective level, as a means of breaking cycles of violence, is ineffectual if not altogether illusive.

Mourning is a different psychological process from how trauma is survived and managed. Mourning is bound to the loss of a loved object and necessitates a change in an internal object relation. In the experience of genocide, while survivors must mourn family and friends who have been killed, they are also left to manage the trauma of witnessing a world in which violence has had no limits and in which the social norms that allow us to coexist have been demolished. The principal trauma for the survivor is the brutal destruction of an illusion of safety in which basic trust between people prevails. The distinction is an important one. Mourning is in itself a process of recovery that enables the individual to separate from the dead, to survive loss and to form new emotional attachments. It is not possible, however, to recover from trauma in the same way, if at all. It involves much more than accepting loss. It requires us to accept destructive forces, in others and in ourselves, that threaten not only our physical wellbeing but our very sense of who we are as persons. In mourning, our identity is temporarily fractured because of the loss of a relationship that has in some respects defined us. In trauma, identity has been rent apart and is irrevocably altered.

For those who have survived and witnessed extreme violence there is the danger of a breakdown between fantasy and reality. In order to protect itself from psychosis, it is necessary for the ego to reject what Freud referred to as an "unbearable representation" together with its affects. The reality of the traumatic event cannot be fully remembered; its repression enables the ego to restore some kind of cognitive coherence that provides predictability and a sense of safety. What is essentially the mental disavowal of trauma is also entangled with guilt and shame, the guilt of survival itself and the shame of identification with the aggressor. However, even when the reality of the trauma can be validated or witnessed and the need for disavowal mitigated, the rupture created by trauma can never be fully healed. Trauma, whether experienced by the individual or the group at large, can never be "worked through"; it never heals completely and in the case of groups it continues to be re-enacted, especially at times of threat or stress. While the traumatized group may be able to mourn the loss of loved ones and of life before extreme violence, it cannot mourn the experience of trauma itself.

Perhaps the most ambitious example of an attempt to enable collective mourning took place in Rwanda in the aftermath of the genocide. Under the auspices of UNICEF, Dr Colin Murray Parkes, a British psychiatrist and founder of the international hospice movement, spent nine months in 1995 advising President Kagame's government on its path of recovery. Parkes noted various obstacles to mourning during the time he spent in Rwanda. These were the cultural repression of emotion amongst men especially, both amongst the Hutus and the Tutsis, the complete breakdown of law and order that had undermined trust in leaders and the government and created extreme anxiety within the population, a history of tribal and colonial violence that fostered ethnic hatred, and a culture of male initiation rites that centred around violence.[1]

Parkes reported that at a conference he had been invited to attend in Rwanda on traumatic grief there was a general consensus amongst government representatives that the people most in need of psychological help were women and children. This assessment seems consistent with a culture in which men are expected not to show emotion; the experience of trauma is then evacuated by further violent action. Parkes comments:

> None of the Government representatives to whom I spoke seemed to think that it might be men, soldiers and the leaders on both sides, who were in need of help. Yet genocide is not caused by weak women and children, it is most often caused by powerful men. Maybe we need to consider how psychological support can be given to men, and particularly to people in positions of leadership on all sides, who carry a great burden of responsibility and are subjected to great pressure and stress.
>
> (Parkes, 1995, p.7)

While Parkes was primarily focusing on providing individual psychotherapeutic services within both communities of victims and perpetrators, he asks the obvious question, "When it is not an individual but a whole society that is traumatised what responsibility do we have to protect one group of people from another? Can there be a healer of nations, a doctor to treat National Grief?" (Ibid.). Parkes has no answer to this but was acutely aware of the volatile political situation in Rwanda and the challenge of establishing peaceful coexistence amongst a population that had been mortally pitted against each other. Parkes writes:

> In Rwanda the rule of law has broken down. People no longer sleep securely in their beds at night. Neither their own government nor the United Nations were able to protect them from the most appalling horror imaginable. They know that it could happen again and it probably will.
>
> In Refugee Camps in Rwanda and in the surrounding countries, we have millions of Hutu people who have been driven out of their homes by armed members of a tribe whom they have been taught to see as "cockroaches". On the other hand we have millions of Tutsi whose neighbours turned against them to rape and murder them and whose survival today depends on the troops who invaded their country and stopped the holocaust. They know that the forces that are being built up against them are strong and they want to believe that the rest of the world will prevent another holocaust. But their experience of the last leaves them in doubt.[2]

The present Government in Rwanda achieved power by force of arms rather than by democratic process. So did the Government which it overthrew. Democracy can only work if polarisation is not so great that opposing sides destroy each other. At the present time the imposition of democracy in Rwanda would only aggravate the existing tensions between the tribes and run the risk that the majority tribe, the Hutus, would again attempt to wipe out the minority. Even the Arusha Accord, which seemed to provide a possible solution when it was propounded, has been overtaken by events. The road to democracy in Rwanda is likely to be a long one.

I am no lawyer but I imagine that the legal situation in Rwanda is a minefield. Not only has the rule of law largely broken down but it seems likely that big problems will arise when it is re-established. Thus, if everyone guilty of the crime of genocide, the deliberate attempt to exterminate another race, was to be tried and convicted, it is possible that large numbers of Rwandans would be found guilty. It is hard to see what form of punishment would be appropriate.[3] If, on the other hand, an amnesty were to be agreed then the killers would again have got away with murder.

(Parkes, p.10)

Bearing in mind that Parkes was writing only a year after the end of the genocide, he describes clearly some of the extreme difficulties in restoring peace and trust in a government able to assure the protection of the law. It is not surprising that Kagame's autocracy has been successful in holding Rwanda together and in creating the conditions in which its economy can flourish. Because of this, it is hard to imagine that old grievances will not re-surface as soon as there is a crack in government control, most likely when Kagame's rule ends.

Despite this gargantuan effort to assist a nation to mourn, at the end of Parkes's work in Rwanda it was not evident that this had been achieved, or could have been achieved, and Parkes himself, in his final conclusions, pointed to the fundamental importance of restoring rule of law above any other measures of resolving conflict. Parkes concluded that special services should be provided for individuals who had been traumatized but this in turn leaves open the question, who was *not* traumatized in the genocide? It also assumes that if all the individuals in a traumatized society are given therapy and helped to live with and manage their trauma so they can function better in their lives, then the community as a whole will benefit. But here again we find an elision between individual and group behavior. We have evidence every day in our lives that individuals may say and act in one way but may change their behavior and their beliefs radically when they are part of a group. From his experience in Rwanda, Parkes was in fact the first to admit that the idea of collective mourning was a myth and the idea that collective mourning was necessary to break the cycle of violence only compounded this myth (Parkes, Personal communication).

Because the effects of trauma remain embedded in the group, mourning, if it occurs at all, does not put an end to conflict nor does it relinquish grievance. On the contrary, in certain circumstances mourning of the group's losses can serve to unify the identity of a group so that hostilities against the "other" are strengthened rather than mitigated.

The traditional rituals for healing trauma vary across cultures but share the common characteristic that they demarcate the past from the present and aim to restore a world order that has been ruptured. These are often cleansing rituals that are intended to eliminate malevolent spirits, to restore the community to order and leadership, and to reintegrate individuals within the community. While belief systems differ, the purification of the group by acknowledging past trauma is vital in drawing a line under the past so that the group can move towards social reconstruction. In the face of extreme violence and genocide, there has been so much damage to the community that these rituals lose their meaning and become either ineffectual or impossible. Alcinda Honwana points out in the case of Mozambique after the end of civil war:

> In communities where people were killed by their neighbours, where families were divided for long periods of time, where people can no longer muster the resources necessary to carry out the ceremonies properly, and where the reputation of the traditional leaders was compromised during the war, the effectiveness of customary remedies has come into question.
>
> (Honwana, 2006, p.80)

The argument in favor of supporting such customary traditions is primarily that they facilitate social cohesion, for example, by reinforcing spiritual connections with ancestors and re-establishing moral order and a sense of meaning. This also goes some way in explaining the growing popularity of religious fundamentalist groups in Rwanda, the DRC, and other war-torn countries. However, trauma on such a large scale cannot be "forgotten" through such rituals. As Colin Murray Parkes suggests, what may be far more important in healing trauma is the restoration of a degree of security in the form of social order and authority, and a functioning local economy.

Atonement

On 7th December 1970, German Chancellor Willy Brandt spontaneously fell to his knees at a commemoration of the thousands of Jews who had lost their lives in the Warsaw Ghetto. Brandt's act of atonement became a political icon of the twentieth century, the first national acknowledgement of blame that had been made in front of the survivors of the Holocaust and the world. The fact that it was an apparently spontaneous act made it even more moving; it was an act of the heart and seemed neither politically motivated nor manipulated,

For the victim of violence, the only act that can salve the desire for revenge is for the perpetrator to acknowledge the harm done and in this way to seek atonement. Accepting blame, when that is possible, may be enough in itself at least to bring victims and perpetrators together on common ground. Whether or not this can lead to peaceful conflict resolution and reconciliation is a separate question. Brandt's gesture was not only important because he symbolically accepted the mantel of blame on behalf of his country, it was important because it conferred respect to the victims; through this act the victims were recognized as equal human beings who could no longer be relegated as the "other". This recognition given to the victim is fundamental to apology. In June 1997, at the end of Sierra Leone's brutal civil war, Eldred Collins, chairman of the RUF (Revolutionary United Front Party), broadcast an apology: "We looked at our brothers and killed them in cold blood, we removed our sisters from their hiding places to undo their femininity, we slaughtered our mothers and butchered our fathers" (Mitton, 2015, p.25). Collins openly acknowledged murders and violence that could not be denied or ignored; he set the record straight and in so doing established the basis for dialogue in order to prevent further conflict. Nevertheless, behind the scenes, in anger against the politicians whom he felt had betrayed his party during the conflict, Collins also denied many of the abuses levelled at the RUF (Ibid., p.24).

Other world leaders have followed Brandt's memorable gesture with nuanced degrees of culpability and atonement. Queen Elizabeth, in a historic speech in 2011 in Dublin, admitted the "sad and regrettable mistakes of Britain's troubled relationship with Ireland." The Queen addressed those who had suffered and extended her "sincere thoughts and deep sympathy". Although this was not an outright apology, it was the first public acknowledgement that the British had made mistakes, and was welcomed accordingly. The Queen's admission, phrased as regret over mistakes made, was careful to avoid the accusation that the British had no right to be involved in Northern Ireland in the first place.

Five years later, on a visit to Hiroshima, Obama spoke out against the nuclear devastation. Obama implicitly defended the US decision to attack Hiroshima by notably failing to apologize. Prior to Obama's visit, the White House had made it clear that he was not there to apologize or to revisit US actions but to emphasize the global need to deter nuclear war. There were deep splits within the US about the bombing of Japan. President Truman, who made the decision to drop the bomb, later reflected, "I have no qualms about it whatever." Eisenhower, who became Truman's Army Chief of Staff, wrote in a 1963 memoir, "Japan was already defeated … and dropping the bomb was completely unnecessary" (Wright, 2016). However, Obama stated clearly,

"It's important to recognize that in the midst of war, leaders make all kinds of decisions, it's a job of historians to ask questions and examine them ... I know, as somebody who's now sat in the position for the last seven and a half years, that every leader makes very difficult decisions, particularly during wartime."

On the part of the Japanese, the Abe administration, while acknowledging past apologies made by the Japanese government for their actions during the war, also emphasized that future generations should not be accused or made to apologize for the actions of their forebears (Reuters, 2016). What is striking about the US and the Japanese stated positions at this time is that both nations admit that mistakes are made during war and, most importantly, that these mistakes are not within the realm of responsibility of subsequent generations. In other words, a line is drawn in history marking the past from the present and guilt for the past (at least in the instance of war) cannot be maintained.[4]

More recently, leaders from other countries, in an attempt to set the record straight, have made public declarations relating to their colonial past. In May 2021, speaking at the Kigali Genocide Memorial in Rwanda, President Macron of France, stated that his country had not done enough to prevent the slaughter of some 800,000 Tutsis and their Hutu sympathizers and admitted that "France bore heavy and damning responsibilities." He added that France had "a duty to look history in the face and recognise the part of suffering it inflicted on the Rwandan people by keeping silent for too long." Macron was careful to stress that, while France had made mistakes, it was "not an accomplice" to the genocide, pointing out, "the killers who stalked the swamps, the hills, the churches, did not have the face of France" (Wagner, 2021). Macron was setting out the historical facts, acknowledging France's shortcomings, and clearly demarcating the limits of France's responsibility – and guilt. Macron's speech was undoubtedly a peace offering to Rwanda after years of diplomatic rancor and intended to draw a line under the past. As one genocide survivor stated, "What we realised in the speech (Macron) made, you can feel compassion, and you can feel the willingness to actually correct the errors of the past" (Pilling & Schipani, 2021). While Macron's political gesture may have had a conciliatory effect, at least with some groups, it also reads as a non-liability statement (Wagner).

Similarly, Belgium's King Philippe, on his first trip to the Democratic Republic of Congo since assuming the throne in 2013, expressed "deep regrets for the wounds of the past", referring to Belgium's brutal colonial rule. To mark the occasion, King Philippe handed back a traditional Kakuungu mask "on indefinite loan" to the Kinshasa Museum. The mask had been part of a collection of 84,000 Congolese objects belonging to the Royal Museum for Central Africa in Belgium; its return signifies pending legislation for the restitution for these artefacts, seen as part of a process of reparation. But recognition of wrongs does not amount to the same thing as an apology. As Congolese-Belgian activist, Mona Pembele, referring to King Philippe's acknowledgment, stated,

> It is a beautiful speech with regrets and an admission of the misdeeds linked to colonisation and its consequences which still persist today as racism. If we really want to start a relationship of equals, start all over again, they must first apologize.
>
> (Schipani, 8th June 2022, Financial Times)

Apology from the victim's point of view is considered a pre-requisite for equality as it imputes responsibility for past actions, but this is precisely what is not possible for subsequent generations who played no part in these events and who, because of this, are not in a position to apologize or to heal past wounds.

At the same time as Macron was declaring France's responsibility in Rwanda, Germany's foreign minister, Heiko Maas, was recognizing responsibility for the genocide of the Herero and Nama people in 1904–1907 in what was then the German colony known as Namibia. President Hage Geingob of Namibia accepted the apology from Germany along with an offer of billions of euros to fund projects in Namibia. The Hereros objected to this deal, however, calling it "an insult" because it did not include payment of reparations. Nor had the Hereros been consulted. Agreement was reached for German funding of 1.1 million euros for development projects that will directly benefit the genocide-affected communities. This final agreement took five years to negotiate and, as the historian, Kim Wagner, points out, was the outcome of "various financial and geopolitical considerations." The German apology, as with many other countries, served as a conduit to "settle political deals, not historical facts" (Wagner, 2021).

Wagner warns us not to take national apologies at face value but to recognize the political context in which they are made and the motivation to silence calls for restitution. It is notable that in the case of Namibia, as elsewhere, it is the nation responsible for the crimes committed that sets its own terms for atonement. In the case of Namibia, the Germans not only determined the amount of reparation but how it was to be spent. Wagner writes:

> Former colonial powers, it seems, will say anything short of admitting that the imperial project may not have been so progressive after all, since doing so might undermine their national myths of exceptionalism. That is also why such statements tend to focus on the episodic rather than the systemic. Germany is prepared to own up to the Herero and Nama genocide, but is notably silent on the far deadlier suppression of the Maji Maji uprising in German East Africa, which took place at the same time and resulted in as many as 200,000 to 300,000 killed. Historic apologies

are an effective way of controlling the narrative. As historian Tom Bentley has argued, "[they] function as less of a platform of self-flagellation than one of self-congratulation."

(Wagner, 2021)

In his preface to Dostoyevsky's *The Brothers Karamazov*, Freud also describes the shadow side of penance, writing, "… the invading barbarians who killed and then did penance, penance thus becoming a technique permitting murder." Freud identifies the perverse aspect of atonement that allows the sinner to become righteous and then to continue to commit sins under the banner of righteousness or as "progressive" measures. We are seeing today in those countries that have publicly made atonement for the persecution and killing of racial groups, e.g., Germany, South Africa and Rwanda, a resurfacing of racial hatred and xenophobia. This brings into question not only the efficacy of public atonement as a form of moral cleansing and as a preventive to future violence but whether it is in fact morally authentic or appropriate within the context of large group dynamics. While it is important to uphold a certain moral code within society and to restore a belief in justice, collective gestures of atonement and memorialization may create a false sense of unification that can prevent governments from seeing old conflicts re-emerge. Atonement does not by itself protect against the return of the repressed, and in bolstering the idea of atonement as a final settlement it deludes us into a false sense of closure.

There is a further caveat regarding gestures of national atonement that needs to be considered as it is often used to settle the historic "facts", or narrative, of what has happened. In a response to Wagner's article on apologies, Edward Clay, former British High Commissioner of Uganda (1993–1997), Rwanda (1994–1996) and Kenya (2001–2005), points out that imperial authorities are also liable to "confused thinking, which led them into occasional error and excessive violence" (Clay, 2021). Clay's point is also, of course, just as true in warfare or in most political arenas for that matter. Events are not always the outcome of clear decisions and determined policy and, moreover, the "facts" constituting events are not always known. We cannot be reminded enough that even our individual memories are selective in what it is we can and choose to remember.

Rather than expecting acts of atonement to set the record straight and to bring about resolution of past conflict, we might be better off recognizing their limitations and manipulations, and valuing them as a tool towards establishing some form of what Clay refers to as a "modus vivendi" between former enemies. In the case of colonialism, there is, however, a hidden drawback in emphasizing the importance of atonement as a way of establishing equity between the former subject and colonizer. The Algerian novelist and writer, Kamel Daoud, refers to the Stora Report of 2021, commissioned by Macron to promote reconciliation between France and Algeria following 132 years of harsh occupation. Daoud warns us that the importance placed on repentance for past crimes is not helpful in understanding the bonds of domination that continue to influence Algerian society. He writes:

> Focusing exclusively on the sins of the coloniser fixes the colonised in a state of perpetual victimhood. But this remains the approach of western academics, intellectuals from former colonies now residing in the former colonising state, and of elites in the former colony, who exploit the colonial past to further their own interests.
>
> But being a "victim" prevents us from seeing how the memory of colonisation is manipulated by political and economic elites in former colonies, who lay claim to the legacy of the revolution. The west sees the world through its guilt, as it once saw it through its desire for domination. Guilt may be harmless, but it prevents understanding, which is needed for both parties to move forward.
>
> (Daoud, 2021)

Daoud makes the subtle point that the West's desire for domination has morphed into what we can call neo-colonial guilt that enables it to maintain moral and political superiority and to reinforce the bond of domination. The act of atonement, rather than resolving injustices from the past, becomes a means to suppress further grievance while retaining, at its extreme, certain economic and financial control with respect to future development; colonized and colonizer remain in fixed positions.[5]

The Stora Report, criticized and misunderstood by many, has fueled renewed animosity about the past and, as Daoud argues, diverts Algerians from focusing on what they want to make of themselves in the future and of having an identity that is no longer that of the colonized victim.

Letting Go of the Past

In working with individual patients who have suffered extreme forms of abuse, there are certain emotional processes that are necessary to experience before they are able to "work through" their trauma. These processes include having a witness to validate what has happened to them and their experience as victims, being able to hate their abusers without turning that hatred onto themselves, not feeling that they have to forgive their abusers, and being able to accept that what has happened to them cannot be undone. These different aspects of working through trauma do not necessarily follow in a sequential order but are layered and come in and out of consciousness at different times. The final, and most difficult aspect of recovering from trauma of any kind is to be able to dis-identify with it, to regard it as an event that has scarred one's life but has not determined the future and, specifically, one's identity.

One patient, Henry, a successful businessman close to retirement, came to see me because he had a crippling blow at work a few years before and could not stop thinking about it to the point that it was debilitating. Henry was a conscientious, hard-working and intelligent company leader who had been pivotal in building the success of the company he worked for. In a board coup, Henry was suddenly fired just at the point when the company was going to go public. Henry said this was a ruthless and greedy act by a few at the top of the company and it had effectively robbed him of the fruits of his labor for many years, not only financially but in terms of his reputation. The coup was especially painful as it resonated with a family trauma that Henry experienced as a young child. Henry spent many sessions venting his fury with his ruthless colleagues and with his parents whom he had felt similarly used by.

After some time and several failed attempts to recover the position Henry had expected to have in his professional world, Henry began to accept his loss and to find other work that was rewarding. It soon became clear that these new successes could not compensate for Henry's loss; he held on to his grievance with his former bosses like a dog chewing at a bone. We talked about his thirst for revenge, his envy of his bosses' subsequent success, and his earlier anger and disillusion with his parents. He continued to gnaw at this event in his mind. I pointed out that Henry seemed to need to keep an emotional attachment to these selfish and ruthless parents and wondered why this was so important to him. Henry reflected on this and said, "This is who I am – a failure no matter what I set out to do, no matter how hard I try." In saying this, Henry could see how much the early trauma in his family compounded by his subsequent work trauma had shaped his perception of himself – his identity. While as a child, considering himself as a failure was a way for Henry to protect himself from being aware of his parents' failure towards him, this deeply held belief was preventing him from taking pleasure in his actual successes and allowing himself to exert a healthy ruthlessness in his own business dealings. Henry added that he had spent his life fighting against the threat of failure, a failure that had in fact already happened but which continually haunted him in the present. He explained that "giving up" on this fight had always felt very dangerous, that it would be a relinquishment of power and leave him truly helpless. Carrying on the fight, at least in his mind, was Henry's ongoing battle not to be defeated as he was in reality. Henry gradually became more aware of how much these traumas had shaped his identity and how frightened he was of no longer seeing himself as a failure and a victim. After reading about another success of the company that had fired him, Henry felt a pang of fury and then stepped aside in his mind realizing that he didn't actually care about them or about wanting revenge anymore. He admitted in his next session that it had been his desire for revenge that had kept him attached obsessively to the point that it had nearly ruined other things in his life, including new work opportunities.

Another patient, Joseph, a middle-aged man in political exile from his country of origin, had a similar struggle in separating from his country and from the leader who had sent him into exile. For a few years after settling in the UK, Joseph's feelings fluctuated between depression and anger. Everything he had in his life, his work, his public position, his family, his friends, his home, had been taken away by force. In his fury, Joseph said he would never be "at home" in the UK, or anywhere else, because that had been stolen from him. As Joseph gradually did settle into his new life and was able to mourn his losses and to imagine a different future, he would at the same time revert to being the victim once again who had no agency and no future. These times of self-pity were usually triggered by frustration, as if he used the frustration to reinforce a familiar view of himself as a helpless victim while it was also a way of blocking off any thoughts of a positive outcome that would sever his attachment to his tormentor. As long as he saw himself as the victim he kept his tormentor alive in his mind and, at an unconscious level, was declaring to the world, "Look what you have done to me, you have ruined my life."

These individual examples are merely snapshots of the psychological bonds that often remain in place between victim and perpetrator, that maintain this relationship but most importantly that continue to constitute an identification of self as the victim, tainted with the mark of abuse forever. Being able to see how this has been shaped and has formed an integral part of one's identity, especially in cases in which there has been earlier trauma, is vital in enabling the individual to begin to see himself differently and to form new attachments and a different narrative of the self. When we encounter people who hold grudges against their enemies, we are immediately aware of how much their hatred is defining them but also how impenetrable they are to any other experience in the present. The grudge becomes a perverse defense that maintains a relationship of hate and revenge.

Dr Colin Murray Parkes, after his work in Rwanda, questioned how it is possible to provide therapy to a whole nation. Even if therapy was available to every individual, what, if any, difference would this make to the nation as a whole and how it relates to its past? What difference would it make to how we use blame and guilt to define ourselves and others? These questions take us back to the difference between the nature of individual identity and group identity. While our individual identity needs to be plastic in order to ensure that we conform and survive within the group/s we belong to, a group's identity, particularly when it is under threat, is defined to a large extent in relation to the "other" or the enemy. Perhaps, as in the case of Henry and Joseph, a large group cannot risk giving up its enmity without at least the fear, if not the reality, of being extinguished altogether. We can see this dynamic at work in many of the intransigent, long-standing political conflicts across the world in which years of unrelenting animosity and violence seem to have created and reinforced national identities centerd on this conflict.

We have seen in some countries, such as Germany and Rwanda, following genocide, that their current national identity has been bolstered, if not founded on, their acknowledgement of guilt and the measures that have been taken to atone for their crimes. As Daoud warns, however, to what extent has guilt been used as a trump card in establishing a neo-colonial position *vis a vis* other countries? The guilty countries are the ones who rule now, as they have before. On the other hand, there are the countries that remain seemingly stuck in the feuds and grievances of their past; blame has become an integral part of their identity. While those countries that accept guilt seem to have the upper hand in furthering their own interests, the countries that are tied to blame seem to be caught in a perverse mutually destructive relationship where there is no future.

A tragic example of the cycle of blame and denial can be seen in the ethnic and nationalistic identity hostilities that continue to be enacted in the small mountain town of Srebrenica in the easternmost part of Republika Srpska, an entity of Bosnia Herzegovina. During the Bosnian War, in July 1995, following the withdrawal of UN Dutch peacekeeping forces from what had been designated as the safe zone of Srebrenica, Bosnian Serb forces under the command of Ratko Mladić took control of the area, slaughtering more than 8,000 Bosnian Muslim men and boys. The massacre was subsequently recognized by the International Court of Justice (ICJ) and the International Criminal Tribunal for the former Yugoslavia (ICTY) at The Hague as genocide perpetrated by the Bosnian Serb army with the support of the Republika Srpska government. Despite these rulings, denial of the genocide amongst Serbs and Serb-dominated parts of Bosnia has been promoted and has increased significantly. Bosnian Serbs accept what happened as a crime but not as genocide, emphasizing that there was no intent at ethnic cleansing. Since the genocide ruling was made, both Radovan Karadžić, the Bosnian Serb leader, and Ratko Mladić have been convicted of genocide and sentenced to life imprisonment by the International Criminal Court at The Hague. Both continue to be hailed as heroes by the Bosnian Serbs. Although there was legal provision in the Dayton Peace Accord of 1995 to criminalize public denial of the genocide, this was only introduced as law in July 2021 by Valentin Inzko, the outgoing Head of Bosnia's Office of the High Representative (OHR) responsible for overseeing the implementation of the peace agreement. Fearful of "sowing the seeds" for further conflicts, Inzko explained, "The situation has gotten worse and is now getting out of hand ... Therefore, I believe that it is now necessary to regulate this matter with legal solutions" (*The Guardian*, 24th July 2021).

Twenty-six years after the genocide, Srebrenica presents a deceptively integrated small society with inter-ethnic football teams, community events and a younger generation who claim not to differentiate ethnic identity amongst their friends and peers. But this generation of Bosnian Muslims is also careful about what they talk about with their Bosnian Serb friends. One young woman explains,

> I think they were always scared of my reaction and my truth about what I know and what they don't know ... And, of course, we never

talked about this topic because I don't want to ruin my relationships with anyone.

(Hopkins, 7th August 2020)

At the same time, inequalities are evident between the two ethnic groups. Before the war, over 70% of Srebrenica's population were Bosniaks (Bosnian Muslims). Today, Srebrenica is the only small town in Bosnia and Herzegovina where the population is evenly split. This might seem promising were it not for the fact that Bosniaks are grossly underrepresented in government jobs, the main source of employment in the area. A young Bosniak man has no illusions that there is systemic discrimination but locates this in the governing elite, saying,

> They send a message that we aren't part of society here, that we can never play a role, that we are not welcome … We live together only because of us ordinary people, in whom there is still something good left, despite everything. One might think that it is the current system or policy that promotes such values. No, they only incite evil, as they incited genocide.
>
> (Ibid.)

There is a clear distinction made here between individual relationships that transcend political and ethnic differences and the relationship with the state that continues to implicitly demarcate and act on these differences. And yet, in introducing a law to prevent the denial of the genocide, Inzko explicitly stated that it was aimed at individuals, not at nations. Inzko stressed the importance of recognizing individual guilt as a means of allowing people to let go of their past and to create a better future (*The Guardian*, 2021). The problem, as we have seen elsewhere when neighbors turn against each other in mortal enmity, despite previous amicable co-existence[6], is that it is the group and its leaders that determine enmity, racial belonging, and, ultimately, survival; it is not the individual.

The racial hatred that is being fomented by the Bosnian Serbs and Serbia is nothing new and harks back to the fourteenth century when Bosnia was taken over and ruled by the Ottoman Empire. When Srebrenica fell to the Bosnian Serbs on 11th July 1995, Mladić declared on camera, "We give this town to the Serb people as a gift", making it clear that the massacre was in "revenge against the Turks." The term "Turks" is used today as a derogatory slang for Bosniaks. Mladić was marking both the Serbian historical "chosen trauma" and its "chosen glory" in this statement of ethnic justice and moreover of Serbian ethnic identity.

The war of revenge continues to this day; responding to the 2021 ban on genocide denial, Milorad Dodik, the leading Bosnian Serb politician and outspoken nationalist described Inzko, the proponent of the ban, as "a foreigner who will destroy Bosnia, he is taking revenge on Serbs and Croats"

(Hopkins, 4th January 2021). As the newly appointed Head of the Srebrenica Memorial Center in Potočari and survivor of the genocide explains, "What we have here is a war for the interpretation of the war ... One is factual and based on DNA evidence (referring to the exhumation of bodies) ... The other is based on myths that were based on more myths" (Ibid.). Myths, however, tend to be more powerful than facts because they are the stories of our origins and, as such, define who we are and our place in the world. Myths establish our family or tribal identity and connect us to the gods, whereas facts may be piecemeal and therefore often hard to decipher. Myths enshrine a group's "chosen traumas" and its "chosen glories" and establish a group's purity; the "other" is always to blame. The Albanian novelist, Ismail Kadare, notes, "Blood flows one way in life and another way in song, and one never knows which flow is the right one" (Kadare, 2011).

The Dayton Accord of 1995, while it has quelled violence in the region and achieved a period of peace and relative stability, seems to have done little to ameliorate deep-seated ethnic hatred. And perhaps this is too much to expect in a country that has had centuries of ethnic hatred lived out in unrelenting cycles of revenge and violence. Valerie Hopkins, who reports extensively on Srebrenica, writes that Western media continually ask about the possibilities for reconciliation. Hopkins responds: "Maybe they should have asked Ms Karacic, who no longer lives in Srebrenica but in a city three hours away. 'I just can't look at them anymore,' she says, referring to her ethnic Serb neighbours. 'I know they are not all the same, but I cannot socialise with them anymore. We greet each other, but that's it'" (Hopkins, 16th July 2020).

The only closure that may be possible is to let go, to draw a line under the past and, perhaps like the Bosniak woman, to greet one's former enemy, but that's it. Ms Karacic's solution was to move away to a place where she was not reminded daily of past injuries and her own grievance. However, this is not a solution available to everyone. As long as enmity remains on both sides, cooperation can only occur if there are shared vested interests. Even so, we have seen countless instances in which past feuds take precedence over any benefits that may be gained by working together in the present. The reality is that reconciliation of conflict and healing traumas experienced by large groups may not be possible. At most, what may be possible is to establish a peacekeeping truce so that actual violence and further trauma is not experienced by future generations. It may then be possible for these generations to find common cause in economic or political aspirations that may bring about the possibility for a new group identity and transcend past differences.

Kadare, writing about the ancient tradition of blood feud that has beset his country, warns us that it is easy to remember and far more difficult to forget (Kadare, 2017). Is Kadare somehow suggesting that we need to be able to "forget" in order to "move on" without repeating the past? Kierkegaard elaborates, "When we say that we consign something to oblivion, we suggest simultaneously that it is to be forgotten and yet also remembered" (quoted in Hyde, 2019, p.252). We're unable actually to erase or obliterate the past – this would be a denial and repression of reality, of our own history and identity as well as our psychic reality – but we can mark it as done with or consigned to the past. This is true as much for the individual as the group. While acts of violence are, as Primo Levi states, "forever irreparable" (Levi in Wiesenthal, 1997, p.191), how we choose to respond to them is what gives us, as individuals, agency. As Hyde comments, "it is necessary to forget and remember at the same time", explaining that this paradoxical position is what enables us to reconcile ourselves with the past (Hyde, p.252).

Holocaust survivors, when asked about their feelings towards their perpetrators, in seeking some closure on the nightmare they experienced, respond in a variety of ways, from fantasies at one extreme of total revenge to fantasies of complete forgiveness at the other. Both fantasy responses are different ways of trying to eradicate the stain of being a victim through a reversal of helplessness, by assuming the position of determining the other's life. Although forgiveness of perpetrators continues to be a contentious issue,[7] there are numerous cases of individual survivors who have come forward to forgive their perpetrators. Instances of actual revenge, however, both within the camps and post-liberation, are in fact rare and were generally frowned upon by survivors.[8] In addition, prisoners were aware that actual revenge would not really be satisfying as it would not rectify anything. One prisoner admitted "he knew that he could kill the whole German nation and it wouldn't relieve the feelings he thought revenge would relieve" (Gill, 2018, Loc. 2354). The incidence of suicide both within the camps and post-liberation is perhaps a better indicator of revenge turned inward and enacted against the self. For most individual survivors, attempting to lead a creative life has been the driving force in combatting the destructiveness they have been subjected to and in continuing to be at its mercy. As I have shown in my clinical vignettes, this response cannot repair the past but it can achieve some form of closure and satisfaction.

While individuals may have a better chance of closure, especially if they have a relatively benign superego, group behavior, as we have tragically witnessed, can become perverse under powerful leaders that promote violence as a response to injury or threat to group identity. If the impulse for revenge is licensed by the leaders, the group can only repeat the trauma. In addition, the need to sustain hatred of the other may be so embedded in the group's identity that to let this go would seem paramount to the group's extinction. The cycle of revenge that continues to be enacted blocks any form of closure, much less resolution. The problem is not how do we change this, but how can we understand this and what choices can we make in responding to this without further exacerbating or driving underground the hatred that cannot be quenched?

Notes

1 Parkes astutely linked the genocide to tribal rites of passage. He reported, "In warrior tribes the passage from adolescence to manhood often involved an ordeal and/or acts of bravery and violence towards others. Sometimes this took the form of killing your first lion, at other times taking your first scalp or fighting a battle (which was often bloody) against some supposed foe. Often the ritual involved some sort of public degradation or other pain. The rules of justice and fairness were set aside in favour of a more cruel necessity. To be a man was to control emotion and to become brave, tough and, in these special circumstances, cruel." (Parkes, C.M., "Genocide in Rwanda: personal reflections." 19th October 1995, pp.7–8)
2 The Refugee Camps were broken up by the RPF in 1997–8 killing thousands of Hutus in the process. (Communication from Michela Wrong)
3 Security Council Resolution 955, 8th November 1994 established, by a vote of 13 to 1, an International Criminal Tribunal for Rwanda under which charges of genocide could be brought to trial but it did not provide for the death penalty. Rwanda, by chance, was a member of the Security Council, and voted against the resolution on account of this omission.
4 While it is arguable that the nature and degree of responsibility for war crimes can be distinguished from atrocities such as genocide committed under colonial rule, I am treating them as a common entity in relation to the assignation of blame and guilt.
5 As I have argued, in political processes following extreme violence to impose "forgiveness" as an ideal can also be damaging insofar as it constitutes a neo-colonial imposition/act of aggression on the victimized culture with the message that they should no longer be angry or hurt. See Covington, C. (2017). *Everyday Evils: A Psychoanalytic View of Evil and Morality.* Chapter 7. London: Routledge.
6 See notably, Gross, J.T. (2003). *Neighbours: The Destruction of the Jewish Community in Jedwabne, Poland, 1941.* Princeton: Princeton University Press.
7 See Weisenthal's collection of writers on this subject in his book, *The Sunflower.*
8 Gill also attributes the rare incidence of revenge by prisoners post-liberation as due to the conditions within the camps. Gill writes: "Despite the fact that arms were readily to hand in liberated Buchenwald, very few prisoners even wanted to experiment with revenge. The Germans had failed to brutalize the prisoners as thoroughly as they had wished, and that saved them ... 'We desisted not because we were too exhausted to do it; it was simply that we were too decent; enough of our upbringing had remained, despite all the Germans had tried to do; one simply doesn't do things like that.'" (Gill, Loc. 2360)

References

Associated Press (24 July 2021). "It's getting out of hand': genocide denial outlawed in Bosnia." *The Guardian.*
Clay, E. (11 June 2021). *Letter: Establishing truths about imperial rule is a big ask. Financial Times.*
Daoud, K. (24 February 2021). *The west is too obsessed with its colonial guilt. Financial Times.*
Gill, A. (2018). *The Journey Back from Hell: Memoirs of Concentration Camp Survivors.* Sharpe Books. Kindle edition.
Honwana, A. (2006). *Child Soldiers in Africa.* Philadelphia: University of Pennsylvania Press.

Hopkins, V. (16 July 2020). "Srebrenica's wounds remain unhealed after 25 years." *Financial Times*.

Hopkins, V. (7 August 2020). "Inside Srebrenica: old scars, new wounds." *Financial Times*.

Hopkins, V. (4 January 2021). "Old tensions still alive in Bosnia 25 years after Dayton." *Financial Times*.

Hyde, L. (2019). *A Primer for Forgetting: Getting Past the Past*. New York: Farrar, Strauss & Giroux.

Kadare, I. (2011). *Three Elegies for Kosovo*. London: Vintage Classics.

Kadare, I. (2017). *The Traitor's Niche*. London: Harvill Secker.

Mitton, K. (2015). *Rebels in a Rotten State: Understand Atrocity in Sierra Leone*. London: Hurst & Company.

Parkes, C.M. (1995). "Genocide in Rwanda: Personal Reflections." *Morality* 1(1), 95–110.

Pilling, D. & Schipani, A. (27 May 2021). "Macron admits French responsibility in Rwandan genocide." *Financial Times*.

Reuters. (22 May 2016). "Obama will not apologize for Hiroshima attack, he tells Japanese tv". *The Guardian*.

Schipani, A. (8 June 2022). Belgian King regrets 'wounds of past' in first Congo visit. *Financial Times*.

Wagner, K. (4 June 2021). "Apologies for historical atrocities fall short of a formal reckoning". *Financial Times*.

Wiesenthal, S. (1997). *The Sunflower*. New York: Schocken Books.

Wright, R. (12 May 2016). "What the Pope Saw in Hiroshima". *The New Yorker*.

Chapter 8

The "Empire of Lies"

Russia's War in Ukraine

What happens when what you've believed is a lie? Does that make you guilty?

(James, ex-soldier)

Invasion

My discussion of blame and collective guilt would not be complete without an attempt to understand the political dynamics and rationale of Russia's invasion of Ukraine on 24th February 2022. While some Russia experts had anticipated this would happen, it nevertheless came as a blow to Western nations and presented an imminent threat to Eastern European countries that had been within the Soviet bloc and those countries, such as Poland, bordering Russia. The invasion also elicited a certain amount of dismay within NATO countries that Russia's invasion of Crimea in 2014 had virtually gone unchallenged. It had been a wake-up call that had been largely dismissed at the cost of Ukraine's safety.

In his speech marking the invasion of Ukraine, Putin laid out a clear narrative outlining the events that had, in his view, cumulatively, given Russia no choice but to defend itself. Putin's list of Western threats and territorial aggression in Eastern Europe not only provided the justification for Russia's response but described a history of Russian humiliation, betrayal and victimhood – wounds that remain painful in Russian memory. In particular, Putin cites Russia's grievances against deceitful Western governments. Referring to the collapse of the Soviet Union and increasing efforts by the West to encircle and destroy Russia, Putin stated:

> … This array includes promises not to expand NATO eastward even by an inch. To reiterate: They have deceived us, or, to put it simply, they have played us.

Within this narrative, Putin accused the West of supporting separatist groups, such as in Chechnya, attempting to divide and weaken Russia.

DOI: 10.4324/9781003379980-9

This is how it was in the 1990s and the early 2000s, when the so-called collective West was actively supporting separatism and gangs of mercenaries in southern Russia. What victims, what losses we had to sustain and what trials we had to go through at that time before we broke the back of international terrorism in the Caucasus! We remember this and will never forget.

In building his case for the invasion of Ukraine, Putin mounted a series of "false flags" that described a projected cultural and political enemy that must be vanquished in order to preserve Russian territory and "to defend people who have been victims" under Kyiv's regime.[1] Putin went further to claim that it was the neo-Nazis in Ukraine's regime, supported by NATO's leading countries, that were committing genocide on the Russian population. He explained:

> This brings me to the situation in Donbass. We can see that the forces that staged the coup in Ukraine in 2014 have seized power, are keeping it with the help of ornamental election procedures and have abandoned the path of a peaceful conflict settlement.
>
> We had to stop that atrocity, that genocide of the millions of people who live there and who pinned their hopes on Russia, on all of us.

Putin also described the threat that NATO countries "who will never forgive the people of Crimea and Sevastopol for freely making a choice to reunite with Russia," would not stop with Ukraine but would go on to attack Crimea. He predicted the slaughter of "innocent people just as members of the punitive units of Ukrainian nationalists and Hitler's accomplices did during the Great Patriotic War. They have also openly laid claim to several other Russian regions." Putin's words were a forewarning of his own ambitions to recover what were once considered Russian regions.

The most powerful message in Putin's speech is the claim that Russia is facing an existential threat and has no choice but to fight for its identity and ultimate survival.

> For our country, it is a matter of life and death, a matter of our historical future as a nation … It is not only a very real threat to our interests but to the very existence of our state and to its sovereignty. It is the red line which we have spoken about on numerous occasions. They have crossed it.

Putin finally emphasized:

> If we look at the sequence of events and the incoming reports, the showdown between Russia and these forces cannot be avoided. It is only a

matter of time. They are getting ready and waiting for the right moment. Moreover, they went as far as to aspire to acquire nuclear weapons.

They did not leave us any other option for defending Russia and our people, other than the one we are forced to use today. In these circumstances, we have to take bold and immediate action.

As we were soon to discover, Putin's words were prophetic – but prophetic in a paranoid reality, projecting an exaggerated mirror image on to Ukraine and the West of Putin's own intentions and worldview. It has been striking that every announcement Putin has made referring to his predictions of Western aggression have in fact signaled his next moves, as if he is transmitting these in advance not only as a justification for his actions but as a provocation which, if acted upon, would validate Russia's position as the victim.

Blame and Truth

Invasion by a foreign country is profoundly traumatic for any nation and leaves its own trace of vulnerability and fear. The invasions of Russia by the Mongols in the thirteenth century, by Napoleon in 1812, and Hitler in 1941 have left deep scars on the Russian psyche – scars that have made Russia particularly anxious about its survival as a state. Putin's repetitive presentation of Russia as a "besieged fortress" underscores the shame and humiliation of the Russian people. By exacerbating the history of Russian humiliation, Putin fosters Russian identification with the victim and the consequent rationale for retaliation.

When a nation's sovereignty and identity are under threat, it seeks to protect and strengthen itself by keeping alive in its collective memory the "chosen traumas" that mark so much of its history and, inevitably, its identity. Within these "chosen traumas", the archetype of the heroic martyr who sacrifices his life for his Mother country is idealized and used to inspire a vision of recovery and a future as great as the past. Alongside the "chosen traumas" are the "chosen glories" that signify the potency and successes of the past and the imperial glory that can be regained and turned to as a curative revenge for humiliation. "Chosen traumas" are also sites of blame and warnings to be alert to further attacks from foreigners who are not to be trusted.

Blame is a recurring theme in Russian history that speaks to many Russians today. While typically blame is cast or ascribed to the enemy without, there is also a certain tradition of blamelessness within the country that reflects a history of apathy and impotence to effect change. The question, "who's to blame?", first came into common parlance with the publication of Alexander Herzen's novel, *Who's to Blame?*, in 1847. The novel was a social and psychological commentary on contemporary life in Russia – amongst the first literary works of its kind.[2] It depicts three good characters who are destroyed by an array of social causes that were not of their own making. The characters are impotent to influence the events in their lives, as individuals they are merely "a chip of wood floating on a river" (quoted in Grenier, 1995). The overwhelming complexity of the social problems faced by the Russian characters in the novel defeats their ability to act with any self-agency. Herzen's argument suggests that those who have no ability to effect social change, much less evaluate what needs to be done, cannot be held responsible for actions of the state. As the individual, and the group, lack any realizable social responsibility, they are in effect blameless *vis a vis* moral judgment.

While Herzen's citizens lacked the self-agency to act in any meaningful way politically, it is questionable how much self-agency Russians feel they have today. State control of the media is a powerful tool to quell dissent and dissent can have serious consequences in any case. Propaganda, however, does not necessarily induce trust in leadership. Recent research indicates that Putin's manipulation of information and the press is more likely to produce political apathy than actual approval. Distrust of propaganda has a deleterious effect that undermines people's capacity for moral judgment and in turn creates a sense of political impotence.

The political scientist, Maxim Alyukov, maintains that autocratic regimes no longer rely chiefly on physical violent repression to create obedience amongst their populations but achieve this through the ways in which media is harnessed to present conflicting narratives that lead to generalized distrust of information.[3] Alyukov comments, "Instead of making citizens trust regime narratives, propaganda often capitalizes on media distrust. Media trust in autocracies is usually low, because citizens are aware that media are manipulated" (Alyukov, 2022). Rather than making citizens question what information they can trust, the effect of propaganda, especially when conflicting narratives are available, is to create distrust of all media. As Alyukov writes:

> This belief in the propagandistic nature of the Russian state media spills over into questioning the very possibility of objective reporting. Although Russian state media attempt to impose a specific interpretation of the Russia–Ukraine conflict, one of the central messages of these narratives is not "trust our interpretation of the conflict", but instead "you cannot trust any interpretation". This strategy further exacerbates widespread distrust towards the media, which in turn amplifies support for the war. The following passage from an interview with a professed supporter illustrates how distrust towards the media makes the respondent support, rather than oppose, the war: "I cannot say that I support [the war] because I am against the war. But I cannot say that I am against it either because I think that I do not have enough information. The news is just brainwashing people [...] But what I can say for sure is that I will not openly say 'I am against' until [the war] is over. When it is over, we will

discuss it. But now I am a citizen of my country. Let my country finish what it is doing — even without my approval." When no information can be trusted, the respondent defaults to national identity.

(Alyukov, 2022)

Hannah Arendt pointed out that when unquestioning adherence to the party line is expected, regardless of what is true or not, then nothing is trustworthy and no one can make up their minds. It deprives the group of being able to think and judge – and ultimately to act (Arendt, 1967). However, as the Serbian scholar, Vedran Dzihic, argues, bewildering stories and lies "throws dust in the eyes of the public" and can be even more effective in reinforcing the group's subservience to an autocratic leader (quoted in NYR Daily, "The Age of Total Lies", V. Pesic and C. Simic, 6th February 2017).[4]

These findings throw into question the extent to which the Russian population actively supports Putin's war of aggression in Ukraine and what opinion polls are actually reflecting.[5] While younger generations, increasingly urbanized and who have had greater exposure to the West, are more likely to challenge Putin's actions, it is hard to differentiate between others who endorse the regime's narrative and those who remain silent out of distrust. It also raises a more fundamental question about collective responsibility.

The Chosen Myth

The dissolution of the Soviet Union marked the end of communism and socialist ideology. By the time Putin came to power as Prime Minister on 9th August 1999 Russian political ideology was virtually non-existent. The following two decades saw Russia's economy thrive. With increased exposure to the West came increased awareness of civil rights and political freedoms heretofore unavailable. What was notable during this time was the absence of a guiding political ideology or vision of Russia.[6]

The Belorussian journalist, Svetlana Alexievich, in her book *Second-Hand Time* (2013), documents a bitter nostalgia across generations and classes for the political beliefs that had inspired them to live with hardship and deprivation in the past. She writes about the communist vision to remake the

> old breed of man ... Seventy-plus years in the Marxist-Leninist laboratory gave rise to a new man: *Homo sovieticus* ... People who come out of socialism are both like and unlike the rest of humanity – we have our own lexicon, our own conceptions of good and evil, our heroes and martyrs. We have a special relationship with death.
>
> (Alexievich, 2013, p.23)

When it was all over, as one woman complained,

"All of our suffering was in vain ... It's terrible to admit it and even worse to live with it. All of our gruelling labour! We built so much. Everything with our own hands. The times we lived through were so hard! ... After Stalin died, people started smiling again; before that, they lived carefully. Without smiles."

(Ibid., p.141)

And yet, having lived through these hard times, this woman also decried a new world empty of meaning. She said, "Nobody believes in anything anymore. Not in the *domovoi*[7], and not in communism. People live without any kind of faith!" (Ibid., p.139).

Timothy Snyder, a historian, describes the collapse at the end of the Soviet Union of what he terms the "politics of inevitability" that holds the promise of a better future. All the suffering of those years in the name of communism and for what? The "politics of inevitability" was superseded by what Synder refers to as the "politics of eternity". Snyder writes:

Eternity places one nation at the center of a cyclical story of victimhood. Time is no longer a line into the future, but a circle that endlessly returns the same threats from the past. Within inevitability, no one is responsible because we all know that the details will sort themselves out for the better; within eternity, no one is responsible because we all know that the enemy is coming no matter what we do. Eternity politicians spread the conviction that government cannot aid society as a whole, but can only guard against threats. Progress gives way to doom.

(Snyder, 2018, p.8)

With the demise of socialist ideology and a utopian view of the future, we can see how Putin has created a "historic future" that is based on the return of the past and centers around the safeguarding of Russia's identity.

Certainly Putin is no ideologue.[8] Strongly influenced by the Russian fascist philosopher, Ivan Ilyin, and Russian ethnologist, Lev Gumilev, Putin has resuscitated the identity of imperial Russia – of a Russia that harks back to the Mongols and spans the breadth of Eurasia. As Putin announced, "The Eurasian union is a project meant to preserve the identities of nations and the historic Eurasian community in the new century, in a new world." It could be the Soviet Union reincarnate, the significant difference being that alliance rests on the core identification of being Eurasian rather than Soviet. It is not a political union, it is a quasi-spiritual ethnic union binding Russia together. From what was an ideological vacuum, Putin has injected a vision of a mythic past to bolster Russia's ailing identity. This has also enabled Putin to blame his predecessors, Lenin and Stalin, for creating the concept of the Soviet Union that granted a degree of local autonomy that ultimately, according to Putin, caused the schisms within the state that resulted in its break up.

Putin's vision of a Eurasian community encompasses Ilyin's conception of Russia as "an organism of nature and the soul", a virginal nation, "without original sin" (Snyder, p.23). As such, the sovereignty of Ukraine and other territories tied to Russia historically becomes as inconceivable as separating a limb from a body and expecting it to continue to exist. Ilyin denied Ukraine's separate existence, assuming that it would be included in a post-Soviet Russia – acknowledging Ukraine as an independent entity was equivalent, in Ilyin's view, to being a "mortal enemy" of Russia (Ibid.). Prior to Russia's invasion of Ukraine, Putin echoed Ilyin's position, explaining that Ukraine was not a "real" county but was in fact part of Russia, sharing Russia's "own history, culture and spiritual space" (Putin's speech, 24th February 2022). Seen from this perspective, Russia's invasion of Crimea and Ukraine is Putin's attempt to resurrect the empire that Peter the Great had established and to restore Russian purity. Putin's identification with Peter the Great should not be merely attributed to Putin's narcissism; it is a carefully constructed historical analysis that draws on the "chosen glories" of Russia's past to recreate and consolidate a particular "chosen myth". In the absence of ideology, Putin has turned to this "chosen myth" as a means of shaping Russian identity in the present.

Gumilev's influence on Putin and the creation of what I am calling the "chosen myth" has been apparent in Putin's emphasis on nationalistic values of sacrifice and loyalty in order to achieve the restoration of the Russian body. By May 2012, following his re-election as President, Putin had essentially transformed the Russian state according to Ilyin's proposals to create a constitutional autocracy.[9] In his annual speech Putin warned against foreign interference in Russian politics, emphasizing that, "Direct or indirect meddling in our internal political processes is unacceptable" (Reuters, "Putin, in Annual Address, Denounces Foreign Meddling," 12th December 2012). At the same time, Putin stressed the need to preserve "national and spiritual identity". But the real giveaway was when Putin referred to Gumilev's idea of "passionarnost".

> "I would like all of us to understand clearly that the coming years will be decisive," said Putin, hinting, as he often does, at some massive future calamity. "Who will take the lead and who will remain on the periphery and inevitably lose their independence will depend not only on the economic potential but primarily on the will of each nation, on its inner energy, which Lev Gumilev termed passionarnost: the ability to move forward and to embrace change."
>
> (Clover, 2016)

Fifteen months later, in March 2014, Russia invaded Crimea and the drive to incorporate breakaway states back into Russia began, leading to the war in eastern Ukraine. Putin's reference to "passionarnost" is important as it underpins the rationale for these acts of aggression within a spiritual, philosophical framework. The term itself refers to the human instinct manifest in groups to grow and expand, the internal energy of the ethnos, the driving force of cultural, political and geopolitical creation. This meaning conveys the belief that such a drive, because it is instinctual, is therefore natural and not a matter of choice or policy – it is the Russian spirit and indeed the will of the masses. As an instinctual drive, it also necessarily entails suffering, a condition that the Russian people are only too familiar with across centuries of hardship and differing political ideologies. As we see in Alexievich's accounts of nostalgia for Soviet Russia, suffering for a higher cause provides meaning to life for many people and is at the heart of the tradition of heroic sacrifice for the Motherland. While many Russians in the younger generations increasingly question this tradition and Putin's autocracy, the "chosen myth" Putin is expounding resonates with much of the Russian collective experience and psyche.

Through Putin's narcissistic historical lens, Russia is the perpetual victim that has had to struggle continually to protect herself from foreign enemies, to remain pure, and to be true to passionarnost, i.e. to the will of the ethnos. Snyder describes the shift in Russia from a propaganda of "inevitability", promoting the melioristic belief that everything will get better, to that of "eternity", of a nation besieged that must fight for its very existence. Government can no longer aid society or help it to progress, it can only protect society from threats of attack. With the notion of eternity, the idea of history collapses and the collective mentality remains fixed in a timeless paranoid-schizoid position; evil is always external and unceasing, the group always its innocent victim. As Snyder comments, "Progress gives way to doom" (Snyder, p.8). The leader then assumes the role of savior – the one who will rescue the nation through his actions and at the same time absolve the group of responsibility or judgment as this is not needed when the group is by definition innocent.

Collective Guilt?

The war in Ukraine highlights the complexities of applying concepts such as collective responsibility and collective guilt to a nation in which there is not only a certain amount of dissent but the information available through state-censored media is so manifestly distorted. Under an autocratic regime that allows for minimal dissent and in which decision making regarding foreign policy is largely, if not exclusively, in the hands of Putin and his immediate coterie, it is hard to confer responsibility for actions taken abroad on to the Russian population. This is even more difficult when the population lacks trust in the information that is available and, lacking trust, they lack the means to judge.[10] We return to Hannah Arendt's point that without the ability to judge, we have no moral compass and are at the mercy of the leader who determines the truth. Without judgement and without responsibility, there can be no guilt – all remain innocent, free of moral wrongdoing and harm. As Graham Greene wryly comments in his novel, *The Quiet American*, "… you can't blame the innocent, they are always guiltless. All you can do is either control them or eliminate them. Innocence is a kind of insanity" (Greene, 1995, p.216).

Putin's adherence to Gumilev's idea of passionarnost emphasizes the purity and innocence of the Russian people who have been victimized from time immemorial. In the case of Crimea and Ukraine, Russian acts of aggression are projected onto the "other", using false flag accusations in the name of self-defense. As if by sleight of hand, guilt is neatly transposed onto the victim. This schizoid or binary position also infects opponents of Putin's actions who condemn all Russians as morally culpable because of their country of origin. The parallel with Nazi Germany is all too evident. Racism rears its head on both sides in a mirror reflection and disables thinking and judgement. While nations and their leaders do have responsibility for their actions towards other nations and can be held accountable for these, ascribing guilt on to the population as a whole is a moralistic tool that is often just as discriminatory in its nature as the crime itself.

When innocence needs to be upheld so strongly, it can quickly, as Greene observes, tip over into madness and paranoia. While the NATO alliance has taken great care not to escalate the war in Ukraine, particularly in the face of Putin's threats of nuclear attack, it is apparent that Putin is provoking the West to retaliate in order to justify further Russia's position of being the besieged country. This is the classic position of the bully who gains power by accusing his opponent of being the bully. The real threat is Putin's insistence on his innocence, an innocence that must be defended at all costs.

Three days after the invasion of Ukraine and the announcement of sanctions on Russian banks, Dmitry Kiselyov, the host of Russia 1's flagship television news program, announced against a background of film images of Russian strategic missile submarines going out to sea,

> Our submarines are capable of launching over 500 nuclear warheads, which guarantees the destruction of the US and all NATO countries … The principle is: Why do we need a world, if Russia is not in it?

Kiselyov, often called "Putin's mouthpiece", was clearly conveying the message in his broadcast that there is no limit to Putin's resolve to protect Russia, even if it means that Russia goes down with the rest of the world (Homer-Dixon, 2022). Although many view Putin's threats as bluster and attempt to reassure themselves that no rational leader would actually behave in such a self-destructive way, these are dangerous assumptions that do not take account of the cultural tradition which Putin represents and a belief system that inspires suffering and sacrifice for the sake of the Motherland, extending back to the Mongols and across the breadth of Eurasia. Without this cultural knowledge, Putin's vision and his threats do seem irrational and can erroneously be put down to the rantings of a mythomane. But, as the suicidal end of Hitler's Reich has shown us, this view fails to recognize the insanity of collective innocence and the danger it poses to us all.

Notes

1 Putin's narrative of Ukrainian aggression directly echoes Hitler's justification for invading Poland in September 1939. Nazi propagandists accused Poland of persecuting ethnic Germans living in Poland. The parallel with Putin's claim that Ukraine is persecuting its Russian citizens is evident.

2 Gogol's play, *The Government Inspector*, was originally published in 1836 with a revised edition published in 1842 when his short story, *The Overcoat*, came out. Dostoevsky's novel, *Poor Folk*, was published in 1846.

3 Alyukov's argument distinctly focuses on the role of distrust in subjugating citizens. For a detailed description of the move from violent repression to information manipulation as a more effective form of civil control, see Guriev, S. & Treisman, D. (2022). *Spin Dictators: The Changing Face of Tyranny in the 21st Century*. Princeton: Princeton University Press.

4 The effect of media distrust in silencing civil dissent is not only a phenomenon of authoritarian regimes but is also clearly evident in democratic societies, such as the United States, beleaguered with "fake" news.

5 Following the invasion of Ukraine, the Levada Center opinion poll reported an increase in Putin's approval ratings to 71 percent, nearly reaching his highest rating of 79 percent in May 2018.

6 See Chapter Eight in Covington, C. (2021) *For Goodness Sake: Bravery, Patriotism and Identity*. Phoenix Publishing House.

7 House goblin of Russian folklore.

8 A Kremlin consultant claims Putin "hates the word ideology". (Quoted in Guriev, S. & Treisman, D. (2022). *Spin Dictators: The Changing Face of Tyranny in the 21st Century*. Princeton: Princeton University Press. p.75.

9 For Ilyin, the leader and redeemer of the people was a "democratic dictator". Freedom of the individual accordingly meant submission to the collective and subjugation to its leader. (See Snyder, p.47)

10 This is not to say that large groups are not collectively responsible for their actions, but that responsibility is not a categorical concept but contingent on a number of social factors. It is also not to say that democratic societies are more responsible collectively than autocratic societies.

References

Alexievich, S. (2013). *Second-Hand Time*. London: Fitzcarraldo Editions.

Alyukov, M. (2022). "Propaganda, authoritarianism and Russia's invasion of Ukraine." *Nature Human Behaviour*, 6, 763–765.

Arendt, H. (25 February 1967). "Truth and Politics." *New Yorker*.

Clover, C. (11 March 2016). "Lev Gumilev: passion, Putin and power." *Financial Times*.

Greene, G. (1955). *The Quiet American*. London: Vintage Classics.

Grenier, S. "Herzen's Who is to Blame? The Rhetoric of the New Morality." *The Slavic and East European Journal*, 39(1), Spring 1995.

Homer-Dixon, T. (10 March 2022). "Two things the West must do to lower the probability that Putin will pull the nuclear trigger." Cascade Institute.

Pesic, V. and Simic, C. (6 February 2017). "The Age of Total Lies." *New York Review Daily*.

Reuters (12 December 2012). "Putin, in Annual Address, Denounces Foreign Meddling,"

Snyder, T. (2018). *The Road to Unfreedom: Russia, Europe, America*. London: The Bodley Head.

Epilogue
Beyond Blame

Blame arises not just out of injury but out of injustice. It is a reaction that immediately reflects our idea of what is right and wrong, of our innate personal and social morality. Blame is also an acknowledgement that we are responsible for our actions, even when we deny we have done anything wrong or hurtful. We all find it easy to blame others for the injustices of life, more difficult to own up to the harms we commit. As I have tried to show, when it comes to blame, guilt and forms of reparation, groups behave differently than individuals and, more often than not, in ways that disappoint us or that we abhor. We expect groups to behave as we would individually. This is despite the fact that we know what it's like to be swept away by a group and to do things that we might not ordinarily otherwise do.

In trying to understand large group behavior, our first mistake is to apply the moral code we expect of ourselves as individuals to the group. Our blindness to this difference is perhaps rooted in our not wanting to accept the powerful effect of group behavior on our own sense of agency – i.e. that we can go along with actions taken by the group that we would not normally condone – and that belonging to a group is vital to our survival and to our identity. If we lose sight of the important distinctions between what it means to be an individual and what it means to be a group, we will not be able to understand why it is that political conflict recurs, why it is so often irresolvable, and why we don't learn from history.

Cycles of blame can be compared to a game of hot potato; the hot potato is passed back and forth and when it lands unavoidably on one side, there are various ways, as I have described, to lessen its effect, to cool it down. The most effective methods of restoring a sense of justice undoubtedly lie in the public acknowledgement of facts – setting the record straight – and acts of atonement on the part of the nation or group that has harmed others. Even these methods are subject to political manipulation and can be used to serve interests other than justice. What is perhaps more to the point is that at their most effective, these methods alone cannot prevent a resurfacing of old hatreds and blame. The scapegoat is necessary to bind the group together and to cleanse it of its sins. This dynamic is as old as the hills and will not change.

DOI: 10.4324/9781003379980-10

While there is no set formula for breaking cycles of political conflict, there are certain common necessary ingredients to restoring peace. Any attempt to resolve conflict is doomed without an agreed legal framework or set of rules. These ingredients are: 1) recognized and enforced rule of law; 2) leadership that supports rule of law; and 3) the provision of a social space in which conflict can be thought about, expressed, and ameliorated – this is normally the role of government. The emphasis on preserving rule of law is of greatest importance as it is this political framework that establishes safe boundaries for the group and in doing so, a safe means of containing group anxiety so it is not expelled through action but can be thought about and transformed. At the same time these tenets are based on the assumption that rule of law upholds justice, which, of course is a fallacy if it is founded on the interests of the elite or autocratic rule.

Establishing rule of law, at least in its democratic form, is fundamental to restoring justice and in this sense may be the only truly effective way of healing conflict both between and within groups. But law determines what actions are socially acceptable and what actions are not, it does not determine how nations or groups *should* feel. This is the recent territory of psychotherapy as it is applied to political conflict and is most evident in the memes surrounding ideas of forgiveness, guilt, and reparation. There is scant evidence that these ideas of what is morally correct for nations or groups to feel actually work as a way to heal the past. But we want to believe they do. While our dogged belief may be a symptom of denial, as I have suggested, it can also be regarded as a tool of our post-colonial zeitgeist that is as aggressive as the colonial supremacy of the past, cloaked in good intentions. It confers the power of the self-righteous. It is also equivalent to the therapist instilling in patients that they should want to forgive those who have hurt them, they should feel guilty for their sins and they should want to make reparation. These feelings may be helpful for some individuals but they may also be damaging when they do not reflect the patient's reality. This then becomes the colonization of the patient by the therapist.

While it is human to want to blame the "other" for the harm they have done, when it comes to large group conflicts, is it in fact helpful to blame or can it fuel further hostilities? Do we need to find new rituals that are less fixed on laying blame but more effective at peace-keeping; rituals that help us to understand and acknowledge the hatred and violence that has occurred and often continues to exist; rituals that can help us to acknowledge conflicts without acting them out through violence; and, finally, rituals that do not stigmatize a group of people and in doing so create the same mistake as the perpetrators? Do we need to find rituals that bring us together in our mutual shame rather than rituals that tear us apart in guilt? And, as important, can we create rituals that do not heap blanket designations on groups but convey the nuances and real differences that exist within groups that can nevertheless result in mass crimes?

Blame is fundamentally a reaction to loss and the belief that if someone is to blame then the loss can be undone in some way. The function of our belief in a supreme being is that there is some explanation, some game plan, for the pain and losses in our life – and someone to blame, even if it is the gods. Without this belief, we are left to find our own way to acceptance and our own limitations.

V.S. Naipaul eloquently writes:

> … Sometimes in a storm beautiful old trees are uprooted. You don't know what to do. The readiest emotion is anger. You start looking for an enemy. And then you very quickly understand that anger, comforting as it is, is useless, that there is nothing or no one to be angry against. You have to find other ways of dealing with your loss.

(Naipaul, 2011, p.16)

Reference

Naipaul, V.S. (2011). *Magic Seeds*. London: Picador.

Index